Practical Manual of Fetal Pathology

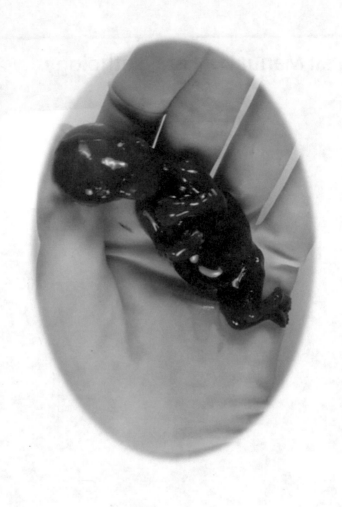

Jelena Martinovic
Editor

Practical Manual of Fetal Pathology

Foreword by John M. Opitz

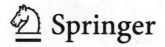

Editor
Jelena Martinovic
Department of Fetal Pathology
Antoine Béclère Hospital, AP-HP
Paris Saclay University
Paris
France

ISBN 978-3-030-42494-7   ISBN 978-3-030-42492-3   (eBook)
https://doi.org/10.1007/978-3-030-42492-3

This Springer imprint is published by the registered company Springer Nature Switzerland AG
The registered company address is: Gewerbestrasse 11, 6330 Cham, Switzerland

Foreword

On a Prefatory Note

Fetoplacental pathology is the last frontier of human biology and medicine given the appalling prenatal death rate of our species (>50%), much of which remains unexplored. By "fetoplacental" I understand the *fetus* from term to 57 days of gestation, the embryo from 56 days to fertilization, and the *placenta* as all trophic tissue at all stages, intact or in pieces, to be sorted from decidua and clots in the lab. And I do so in the hope that all of you are or will be working in services that cover *all* pregnancy stages without sequestering those up to 12 weeks of gestational age as "products of conception" into Surgical Pathology where they may receive only step-motherly attention. And, finally I do so with the expectation and confidence that your place of work is not just a perfunctory service morgue but also an exciting classroom open to any and all advances in developmental biology, pathology, and genetics and a laboratory initiating research in all of these areas toward a better and deeper understanding of human ontogeny. Innumerable causes of prenatal death in humans are yet to be discovered—mutations, TADs, aneuploidies, infections, maternal-placental and epigenetic factors, teratogenic disruptors.

Thus, it is with great pleasure and profound satisfaction that I welcome the Martinovic Manual into life and action. Here is not only a technical *vade mecum* but a biology text by those whose eyes, minds, calipers, and scalpels have been and are guided by insight, decades-long experience, profound knowledge of their subject, and love of their "craft." A beloved, small, but world-renowned band of collaborators in this vineyard, who speak a familiar, universal language, eager to convey wisdom and experience, in practice, to teach, and to urge research. I had a similar experience a half century ago being instructed by an equal master as the Martinovic authors, Enid Gilbert in a 9-year apprenticeship with profound effect on my appreciation of that half of humanity never to nurse or to play with green, plastic dinosaurs. Even before Enid, I had the chance to meet the serious Edith Potter in Chicago: "...put some Prussian Blue on it Opitz!" leading to the discovery of lysosomal defects in Zellweger syndrome. Here I should just say *Vale!* and lay down my pen, but I am tempted to add a footnote on the origin of our discipline.

To this moment in time, developmental pathology has primarily struggled with *morphology*, form and formation, i.e., anatomy and embryology, on gross and microscopic levels, normal and abnormal. Until suddenly, in the 1960s, our vision was marvelously focused and sharpened by *cytogenetics*, the pathology of aneuploidy seen in trophoblastic disease, monosomy X, trisomy-21, -13, -18, triploidy, etc., and the vast amount of *genetic* disease to be seen in CVS samples and POCs alone at, or shortly after the first missed period. So, as cytogenetics barged through the front door of developmental pathology, genetics tiptoed in through the backdoor to become our permanent bedfellow, initially aiding our understanding of gestational *physiology* and *metabolism* with a marvelous array of biochemical and histochemical tests, finally introducing us to *evolution*.

Our field of medicine and biology began very differently from what we now know as fetoplacental pathology, not (yet) as public service but as private instruction, not so much out of the needs of a discipline but of a single person, and not solely focused on humans, but the entire animal kingdom, a perspective we now have lost, sad-to-say. The times could not have been worse—Napoleon had devastated Europe (sort of), defeated Prussia, and occupied Halle closing its University. Nevertheless, Johann Friedrich Meckel Jr. (1798–1862) was able to study in Paris at the *Jardin des Plantes*, beneficiary from the vast natural history collections accumulated under Napoleon and, over 2 years, the collaboration with Cuvier, then Europe's most distinguished comparative anatomist, who, however, disdained evolutionary notions, embryos, and malformations, eagerly taken up by Meckel. His undisputed masterpiece, the *Handbuch der pathologischen Anatomie* (1812), has not been translated into English since 1831. In it, and his voluminous other writings, Meckel adumbrated not only meticulous dissection, preparation, and preservation (a few of his specimens still kept in the Anatomy Department of the University of Halle) but also the notions of:

- Primary malformations as defects of earliest development;
- Malformations as a result of delayed or incomplete ("inhibited") development;
- Multiple segregating anomalies not as coincidences but as causal complexes, in some cases as (now) evident autosomal recessive (Meckel syndrome) and in others as autosomal dominant (the Calleja family of Malta). Thus, Meckel is the father of modern syndromology and clearly knew pleiotropy for what it was;
- Corresponding structures and malformations in humans and other animals as forms of similarity, *analogie*, now homology; wonderful examples are his discussions of unilateral pulmonary agenesis in humans and lung development in "higher" and "lower" snakes; or of Meckel diverticulum as vestigial remnant of the amniote omphalomesenteric duct.
- More yet, Meckel correctly grasped the relationship between the development of the individual and that of the species, i.e., the concept of recapitulation later condensed by Haeckel (1866) into the better-known catch phrase of "ontogeny recapitulating phylogeny."

The fact that during our development we repeat what our direct progenitors and other members of our species have practiced successfully since time immemorial is intuitively obvious. But, repeat how? by inheritance; of what? *die formbildenden*

Elemente (Mendel 1865/1866)—the segregating morphogenetic elements. Elements that are the currency of evolution. Operating how? By natural selection, selection we see daily at autopsy and which has resulted not in what we could have become but what we did become by default—a very frail species indeed. What kinds of *Elemente*? Hereditary units made of DNA (Watson and Crick 1953) to serve as templates for development of individuals through transcription, translation, and replication and of species by mutation. *Elemente* now called genes, biochemical molecules that serve *all* species to resist death, are the basis of *all* organic form and function and, by their very nature, make *all* species more or less vulnerable to extinction and selection. Thus, it is the very same genes that were responsible for the evolution of spiders and of spider monkeys as metazoans, i.e., of animals with epithelia and organs, as the genes that made chimps and humans fellow primates, no supernatural intervention or explanation required.

Finally, we ask: What would paleontology be like without the Meckel cartilage and its evolutionary role in the formation of mandible, TM joint, and middle ear? Just think: trisomy 18 and hemifacial microsomia!

The road ahead for all of us pulling the faculty, student, and trainee wagons together is clear: effective knowledge of human anatomy, embryology, and genetics, and not only knowledge but understanding of the long recapitulatory argument mentioned above. Increasingly we will be receiving lab results stating plainly: mono- or biallelic mutation of gene X at site Y on chromosome Z (HSA or HSX, long or short arm), a sufficient causal explanation if also known or discovered in other "cases" with corresponding phenotype. What the lab test may also indicate in fine print is that gene X is "highly conserved in *C. difficile*, *E. coli*, *C. elegans*, *D. melanogaster*, *M. musculus*," etc.; in other words, it was present in LUCA over three billion years ago and has served life faithfully from prokaryote to eukaryote, from unicellular to multicellular organization, sea to land to air, and chordate to primate. The dead fetus before you, clearly human, unable to have resisted death in form, formation, or function, yet has so much to teach us as apparently successful phylogeny but failed ontogeny. The challenge to you may involve processes billions of years old, knowing for example that some one third of the protein-encoding genes that were present in LUCA 3.8 billon years ago (Weiss et al. 2016) are still present in humans (Martin, pers. comm. 2019).

On that journey, the authors of Martinovic will be your reliable guides.

John M. Opitz
Division of Medical Genetics
Department of Pediatrics
Salt Lake City
Utah, USA

Contents

Part IV   Neurofetopathological Examination

Part V   Placenta

Contributors

Adrian Charles Anatomical Pathology, Sidra Medicine, Doha, Qatar
Clinical Pathology and Laboratory Medicine, Weil Cornell College of Medicine, Doha, Qatar

Ferechte Encha-Razavi Unité d'Embryofoetopathologie, Hôpital Universitaire Necker-Enfants malades, Paris, France

Beata Hargitai West Midlands Perinatal Pathology, Birmingham Women's and Children's Hospital, Birmingham, UK

Jelena Martinovic Unit of Embryo-Fetal Pathology, University Hospitals AP-HP, Antoine Béclère, Paris Saclay University, Clamart, France

Sanjita Ravishankar Perinatal, Pediatric, and Gynecologic Pathology, Case Western Reserve University School of Medicine, University Hospitals Cleveland Medical Center, Cleveland, OH, USA

Raymond W. Redline Perinatal, Pediatric, and Gynecologic Pathology, Case Western Reserve University School of Medicine, University Hospitals Cleveland Medical Center, Cleveland, OH, USA

Neil J. Sebire Department of Histopathology, Great Ormond Street Hospital and ICH UCL, London, UK

Part I

Legal and Ethical Aspects of Fetal Examination Worldwide

Abstract

In no other area of anatomical pathology, does law, ethics, and religion play such a large role than with the mortuary and the autopsy, and pathologists dealing with autopsies, especially those of children, babies, and fetuses, are particularly sensitive, and pathologists need to be aware of the wider legal and social issues involved. Over the last 20 years or so, many national inquiries and investigations have focused on this area, becoming front page news and often leading to similar investigations in other countries. These issues have led to huge distress to the families and professional staff in pathology departments, and sometimes to introduction of new laws, regulations, and codes of practice.

This review is not meant to give current information for every country. The laws and the guidelines from national and international bodies change and society is also changing. The review addresses many areas related to the postmortem procedures in mortuary and fetal/perinatal pathology departments where the law or ethical guidelines impinge on practices and procedures. The chapter has been ordered to cover the workflow through the department from before receipt to release of the body, organs, and tissues.

Perinatal Postmortem Procedures and the Law

Adrian Charles

Introduction

Law, ethical discussions, and religion play a large role in the procedures in the mortuary and for the autopsy, and pathologists dealing with autopsies, especially those of children, babies, and fetuses, need to be aware of the wider legal and social issues involved. Over the last 20 years or so, national inquiries and investigations have focused on this area, becoming news headlines, often leading to similar investigations in other countries. These issues have led to huge distress to the families and professional staff in pathology departments, with loss of established departments of pediatric pathology, early retirements from pediatric pathology, and introduction of new laws, regulations, and codes of practice.

This review is not meant to give current information for every country. The laws and the guidelines from national and international bodies change and society is also changing. The review addresses many areas related to the postmortem procedures in mortuary and fetal/perinatal pathology departments where the law or ethical guidelines impinge on practices and procedures. Many hospitals will have a workflow associated with the deceased, with paperwork including clinical and legal, transfer to the mortuary and any postmortem procedures (medical or forensic examination) and release to the family or funeral director for burial, cremation, or repatriation. The chapter has been ordered to cover the workflow prior to the mortuary, through the mortuary processes and release of the body, tissues, and organs.

The procedures following a death of any person, and particularly a baby, such as grieving, mode of religious ceremony, mode of burial and remembrances vary greatly between cultures. The autopsy and postmortem examination is readily

A. Charles (✉)
Anatomical Pathology, Sidra Medicine, Doha, Qatar

Clinical Pathology and Laboratory Medicine, Weil Cornell College of Medicine, Doha, Qatar
e-mail: acharles@sidra.org

© Springer Nature Switzerland AG 2021
J. Martinovic (ed.), *Practical Manual of Fetal Pathology*,
https://doi.org/10.1007/978-3-030-42492-3_1

accepted in some cultures, but in others regarded as highly intrusive. Cremation is favored in some cultures, allowed in others and not acceptable or provided in other places. The taking of mementoes, picture, hand- and footprints, and lock of hair is routine in some cultures, but any disturbance of the body, and removing a lock of hair, nail clippings and/or taking hand- and footprints is frowned upon in others. The growing recognition of the rights and wishes of the next of kin has caused re-evaluation of these processes, and this will continue.

The organ retention issues arising in the UK [1] and elsewhere [2] also demonstrate the differences between legally permitted historical practices, current societal expectations, and parental expectations. The gaps and lack of clarity in the legal framework for forensic and medical autopsies and the retention of tissue and organs, in the UK led to the Human tissue act, which has, in turn, created further issues. The different perspectives are easier to see in retrospect, from the pathologists focus on performing an examination and identifying the factors of the death, knowing one cannot go back, gathering samples to investigate the causes with new technology, the natural feelings of the parents about postmortem investigations and what is entailed, and also their desires to have answers to the cause of the death, and with a lack of forums for the different groups to discuss the issues and be aware of the issues.

The medical profession has not always been as careful and sympathetic as we could have been. This is a delicate area that needs to be dealt compassionately, thoughtfully, and transparently with careful communication, and pathologists generally are not accustomed to interact with patients. Parents need assistance to make a decision suitable for them both at the time of the loss and later when future pregnancies are contemplated and the causes of the loss are required for management. We need to be working with the parents in this area. Institutions need a general policy and procedure with some room for tailoring to requirements of the individuals concerned, within the law and reason.

Previous government-directed programs like the collection of postmortem bone samples for strontium 90 without consent (indeed government guidance to keep this confidential) [3, 4] and the postmortem retention of the pituitary for growth hormone, (again it appears without consent) [5], also created issues when these practices came to light. Some pathologists also retained large numbers of tissues and organs with the routine nonspecific and brief consent. These show how quickly previous attitudes and good intentioned policies can look dated and thoughtless. Laws in this area may not be very clear, and may lag social changes, but generally give an envelope of practice in a society. As societies change, old practices can seem insensitive, and new laws and practices evolve. Professional practices, procedures, and laws change, sometimes as a result of publicity around an event and the practice of a generation ago is very different. The status of a pre-registerable fetus was legally medical waste, yet it was clear that the parents felt differently, and indeed the different status of fetal and even embryonal tissues for research shows there was a disconnect here for the same tissues with different purposes. In the 1980s and 1990s, pathologists were asked by the government to retain samples for strontium 90 from fetal autopsy specifically without telling the parents, but at the same time pathologists involved in coronial autopsies with requirement to take samples and organs to confirm the cause of death were later criticized for this retention without consent.

The fetal autopsy and disposal of the body, organs, and tissues and the appropriateness of investigation, research, and even the disposal are surrounded by ethical and legal issues. Front page news stories including fetal bodies being discarded with hospital waste, lost, and organs being retained without explicit consent used to be not uncommon. The fact some fetuses are the result of termination of pregnancy also adds to the ethical sensitivities in this area.

Although social practices have changed, the fundamental human feelings one suspects are less changeable. The attitude of 50 years ago, where a stillbirth was not discussed, and mothers often grieved by themselves jars against the number of women who contact the pathology department for any pictures or mementoes (even a microscope slide) up to 30 years or more later saying the stillbirth remains a daily memory. People vary according to themselves, their culture, and their religious beliefs (which may not reflect their inner feelings) in how they respond and remember the baby. In a moslem culture, some of the western practices such as the butterfly sign to indicate a perinatal loss case are regarded as inappropriate, and taking mementoes and disturbing the body especially after the ritual cleaning and shrouding, and the baby is preferred to be buried and soon as it reasonably can.

Gestational age is clearly a continuum, but divided, somewhat arbitrarily by law and practice, such as the gestational age at which a birth is registered, which varies from 16 to over 24 weeks in different jurisdictions. The parents view of their baby though may not vary so much between 18 weeks and 28 weeks despite the change in legal status. A fetus papyraceous delivered at term is often not registered and reactions to an incidental unknown twin who demised in the first trimester but delivered much later is often less an issue.

The laws allowing autopsy also differ in different parts of the world, and in some Islamic countries if allowed at all, medical autopsies are performed only if the cause of death is uncertain. Although religions do not forbid postmortems, it is clear that it is still regarded as relatively taboo or Haram in many. However, this can be addressed in some ethical arguments as a relative issue—cutting a person is haram, but surgery has a greater good, as does the autopsy if the information forthcoming assists the family.

This chapter then will look at different aspects of how the law can affect the postmortem process, from the registration of the birth of the fetus, the role of the legal or forensic autopsy, consent and in some cases authorization of the autopsy examination, retention of organs and tissues, testing for genetic diseases, (and for infectious disease indirectly testing the mother), disposal of the body, and use of tissues for research. The law may affect the place in which a postmortem can be undertaken. As the law is the boundary of practice, it is also important to include ethical considerations. Consent, parental information and procedures must reflect the society in which the death occurs and also the social and religious group the parents may belong too. These may well lead to a more detailed standard of consent and parental information than is strictly required by the law.

Finally, anyone who has worked for long in this area knows the situation is not static, but fluid and the healthcare and the practices must try to remain sensitive to changes in the society in which they operate, and the effect of a headline case may be on practice. Advances such as virtual and minimally invasive autopsy and other technological developments in postmortem investigations may make some investigations easier for parents to accept [6] but more detailed genetic investigations raise other issues. This review is meant to address some of the issues involved, and suggest possible approaches.

Definitions

The law usually defines what cases are subject to that law. However, definitions can be unclear or ambiguous and vary according to the country or even state in which the healthcare operates and sometimes between different laws in the same jurisdiction, leading to gaps [7, 8]. It is therefore important to establish the criteria that may be applied to fetal and perinatal examinations [9]. Common definitions are as below, but need to be checked for the current definition in the jurisdiction under discussion:

1. Embryo
    (a) From conception through blastocyst and development of the inner cell mass, up to the end of organogenesis (around 8 weeks post conception).
2. Fetus
    (a) Generally from end of embryo (~8 weeks post conceptual age) till delivery.
3. Miscarriage (abortion)
    (a) 8–20/24/28 (or registerable age for that jurisdiction) weeks age. Usually not registered officially as a birth, although some countries/hospitals provide a certificate to reflect the delivery.
4. Intrauterine fetal death
    (a) WHO has classed loss at any gestational age, but these are usually divided into miscarriage (or fetal loss, or termination), up to registerable age, whereas stillbirth is over the registerable age. The term can be used differently.
5. Stillbirth registered birth but stillborn
    (a) The lowest gestational age varies from jurisdiction, 16, 20, 22, 24, and 28 weeks are common groups. If the gestational age is unknown, then weight is often used to estimate the age e.g. 500 g for 22 weeks, or 1000 at 28 weeks.
    (b) Sometimes divided into early (20/22–27 weeks) and late (beyond 28 weeks). Late is used more often in developing countries where the early losses may not be so well collated, and for international comparison [10].
    (c) Fetus papyraceous—varies, some jurisdictions state if fetal death in utero occurs early (<20/22/24/28 weeks depending on jurisdiction) with prolonged retention in utero, then the death is not registered [11].

6. Neonate
   (a) Liveborn = Following complete expulsion of the baby, showing movements, breathing movements, and a pulse or heartbeat. This can be for any gestational age in some jurisdictions, but others differ (see below).
   (b) Death = absence of signs of life (brain death is a difficult subject in this group) = No breathing movements, heartbeat, pulsations, movements of voluntary muscles. Some muscular reflex movements or some non-pulsatile movements of the heart or electrical activity are generally not accepted as signs of life. This has been challenged from time to time (see below).
   (c) Viability. Some jurisdictions will certify liveborn babies differently according to the age of viability (<22–24 weeks depending). It is sometimes an issue with very previable fetuses, e.g., <20 weeks, who make some movements, and practices of registration differ [12] as to whether they are captured as live birth or remain fetal losses in official registries.
7. Forensic/Coronial/Legal versus medical examination
   (a) Currently, most stillbirths are regarded as for medical investigation and not for legal (coronial or forensic) investigation as there has been no independent life, and some authorities have argued that there is no jurisdiction for coroners in this area, but other opinions differ (See below).
   (b) One common exception to a medical, non-forensic process for stillbirth is where the birth is unattended by a medical practitioner, nurse or midwife (and often, but not exclusively, when the state of the baby at birth, alive or dead is unclear or uncertain), or a dead baby's body is found. These are commonly referred for a police investigation and medicolegal investigation in many jurisdictions.
   (c) Following suspected illegal abortion.
   (d) A growing area is pressure for medicolegal examination (but is usually not followed) is where the baby is injured and dies in utero or neonatally after trauma by accident or deliberate action or violence against the pregnant mother. The fetal and placental examination though may be used medicolegally in such cases, such as confirming abruption.
   (e) Another area of discussion is making stillbirth examination a forensic process on the principle that as the cause of the stillbirth is often unknown and the routine examination variable, then the same legal approach to unknown deaths in older people is undertaken, and these cases should therefore according to this argument be referred for coronial/medicolegal review to assist in standardizing the examination with the hope of reducing the burden of stillbirths (see below).

References

1. https://www.independent.co.uk/life-style/health-and-families/health-news/forgotten-for-25-years-now-the-1000-infant-bodies-found-after-alder-hey-can-be-laid-to-rest-50417.html. Accessed 2/11/2019.

2. https://www.nytimes.com/2005/08/04/world/europe/discovery-of-stored-fetuses-and-still-borns-roils-france.html. Accessed 2/11/2019.
3. https://www.nytimes.com/2001/10/01/world/british-secretly-used-babies-bones-in-tests.html. Accessed 2/1//2019.
4. http://www.health.sa.gov.au/Default.aspx?tabid=53&mid=449&ctl=ViewDetails&ItemID=85 4&PageIndex=0.
5. https://www.aph.gov.au/parliamentary_business/committees/senate/community_affairs/completed_inquiries/1996-99/cjd/report/c01.
6. Lewis C, Latif Z, Hill M, Riddington M, Lakhanpaul M, Arthurs OJ, Hutchinson JC, Chitty LS, Sebire NJ. "We might get a lot more families who will agree": Muslim and Jewish perspectives on less invasive perinatal and paediatric autopsy. PLoS One. 2018;13(8):e0202023. https://doi.org/10.1371/journal.pone.0202023. eCollection 2018.
7. Nguyen RHN, Wilcox AJ. Terms in reproductive and perinatal epidemiology: 2. Perinatal terms. J Epidemiol Community Health. 2005;59:1019–21. https://doi.org/10.1136/jech.2004.023465.
8. Tavares Da Silva F, Gonik B, McMillan M, Keech C, Dellicour S, Bhange S, Tila M, Harper DM, Woods C, Kawai AT, Kochhar S, Munoz FM, Brighton Collaboration Stillbirth Working Group. Stillbirth: case definition and guidelines for data collection, analysis, and presentation of maternal immunization safety data. Vaccine. 2016;34(49):6057–68.
9. Barfield WD, AAP COMMITTEE ON FETUS AND NEWBORN. Standard terminology for fetal, infant, andperinatal deaths. Pediatrics. 2016;137(5):e20160551.
10. https://apps.who.int/iris/bitstream/handle/10665/249523/9789241511223eng.pdf;jsessionid =E00BA8DE189A09AF3099BF20228897A8?sequence=1.
11. http://policyandorders.cw.bc.ca/resource-gallery/Documents/BC%20Women%27s%20 Hospital%20-%20Fetal%20Maternal%20Newborn/WW.18.08H%20Health%20Records%20 Process%20Death%20Registry.pdf. Accessed 21/10/2019.
12. Mohangoo AD, Buitendijk SE, Szamotulska K, Chalmers J, Irgens LM, Bolumar F, et al. Gestational age patterns of fetal and neonatal mortality in Europe: results from the Euro-Peristat Project. PLoS One. 2011;6(11):e24727.

Death Certification

Adrian Charles

The certificate for a perinatal death is usually completed by the doctor looking after the patient (or mother). Usually, for most ages, if the cause is unknown, or that the case is a legal case, then a death certificate is completed by the forensic medicine team or coroner, after the investigation.

Some jurisdictions have a notification of death—completed the same as above, which is ratified by the governmental authorities before a death certificate and right to burial can occur. This may differ according to whether the patient is a citizen by right of the state or an expatriate.

Live birth certification in many jurisdictions suggests any baby born showing any signs of life should be registered as live born. There are several issues about these definitions [1].

1. In many jurisdictions, the baby needs to be alive when fully delivered. A breech baby who moved legs but is stillborn after delivery of the head is usually regarded as stillborn. The signs of life are usually as above (previous chapter).
2. Some legal authorities have tried to broaden this to include pulseless electrical activity of the heart (see reference); however, this is not in wide acceptance.
3. There are some variations on what is done (and also covered by the law) in extreme preterm—such as 18 weeks gestation, where there is no chance of ongoing life. This has been a particular issue after induction of labor for a severe fetal anomaly such as anencephaly with some movements, and fetal medicine often has procedures to prevent this.

A. Charles (✉)
Anatomical Pathology, Sidra Medicine, Doha, Qatar

Clinical Pathology and Laboratory Medicine, Weil Cornell College of Medicine, Doha, Qatar
e-mail: acharles@sidra.org

© Springer Nature Switzerland AG 2021
J. Martinovic (ed.), *Practical Manual of Fetal Pathology*,
https://doi.org/10.1007/978-3-030-42492-3_2

Care needs to be taken in these cases to know what the local laws are, and the current accepted interpretation, as the laws themselves may not be clear. Institutions involved in this area should have well-considered policies that have been vetted by legal teams and a way to discuss borderline cases. A baby born who does not fulfil the livebirth criteria tary muscle movements etc) will be registered stillborn, if of a registerable age. There may be time limits within which a birth must be registered (e.g., 42 days in the UK, 21 in Scotland). Expatriate babies may get a local birth certificate, but also require a certificate from the parents' homeland for citizenship and visa purposes, and there are laws and procedures associated with this on government websites.

Registerable Stillbirths

Different jurisdictions have different rules. Some have a certificate for stillbirths, and usually no separate death certificate is issued. The gestational age at which stillbirth is registerable also varies, 20 weeks in some countries (e.g., Australia), 24 weeks in others (e.g., the UK), and reflects the current age of viability. This is an area that has been discussed recently in the UK parliament [2]. If the gestational age is uncertain a weight of 400 or 500 g may be used, again varying by jurisdiction. Either can take precedence, but where accurate dating scans are common, the gestational age usually, but not always, takes precedence.

Questions that need to be addressed are what happens if the fetus although of registerable gestational age died well before this age—the extreme example is fetus papyraceous. These are often not registered [3].

It should also be noted that cause of death as unknown is generally not allowed for most death certificates. However, for stillbirths the cause is often unknown (and may indeed be a reason for requesting an autopsy). In many jurisdiction "unknown" cause of death is permitted for stillbirth registration.

Terminations of Pregnancy

This issue is related as it is intricately tied up with the whole area of fetal loss. It involves political and social issues including women (and parental) rights, and reproductive choices. The use of the word abortion for both induced delivery (medical and backstreet illegal), and spontaneous losses, also leads to use of other words, such as miscarriage, stillbirth, and induction of labor. Although terminations are often the result of identifying a serious fetal anomaly, the autopsy performs an important audit and adds additional information for more detailed counselling [4].

The positions are very varied. In some countries with a strong religious influence on laws (for example, Ireland [5]), there may be a strong view against termination of pregnancy for any reasons (including threat to the life of the mother and rape) have been the position until recently. However, recent events have led to a change in the law, including some high profile cases including the death of a woman from sepsis who was denied termination, and some mothers whose human rights were deemed infringed by having to travel abroad for termination after the diagnosis of severe lethal fetal anomalies. On the other side of the world, in Australia in many states abortion was still a crime, jeopardizing obstetricians working in this area. As recently as 2018 and 2019 legislation was passed allowing certain terminations of pregnancy lawful. There are usually strict guidelines and later terminations over 20 or 24 weeks are often more stringent in the procedure to authorize the process with a committee, at limited locations, and also often more stringent conditions of the mother or fetus that need to be met [6]. There are many articles on the law and ethics in this area [7] including the British Medical Association review [8] and a recent review in French compares different countries [9].

In the Muslim world, termination of pregnancy is permitted to varying extents. There is an important religious viewpoint on the ensoulment of the fetus, at 120 days post conception (though this date can vary according to how the Islamic scholar adds together the periods of embryonic/fetal development) which equates to just over 19 weeks gestational age. This does allow good anatomy scans to detect major structural anomalies. However, different Islamic countries have different criteria [10, 11]. A group of experts may permit termination of pregnancy to occur in some jurisdictions.

Forensic and Medical Examination

This is not usually an issue as most stillbirths are medical investigations. However, as stated above there are some exceptions to be aware of, as in many jurisdictions a legal investigation may ensue. The most common situation is a baby delivered with no medical supervision and brought to the hospital dead, especially if there is a history of concealment of the pregnancy, or other complex social issues, and sometimes in the developed world if there is medical care provided by a non-registered "doula."

The other common case is where the babies abandoned body is found. Concealment of pregnancy is a crime in many jurisdictions but in these cases one of the major questions is trying to ascertain signs of life [12]. These may be food in the stomach, inflammation on the outside of the cord, is suggestive of livebirth, (but cord inflammation can be found in chorioamnionitis) and lung aeration is notoriously unreliable [13, 14].

Many jurisdictions have a two or more step forensic process. The possible forensic case can be referred to the police, coronial system, or public prosecutor, whoever is the proper agent. A preliminary investigation may take place possibly involving an external examination, but the autopsy is often a further step. There is usually no consent from the next of kin, though there may be mechanisms for them to object to an autopsy. The coroner or public prosecutor may then direct an autopsy to be undertaken.

Forensic perinatal investigations are complex. Forensic pathologists are experienced in traumatic deaths, but perinatal deaths require familiarity with fetal medicine, scanning, obstetric management, normal fetal development, congenital anomalies, fetal diseases, and placental examination. Perinatal pathologists are likely to be based in the same institution of many of the deaths, giving an apparent conflict of interest in some cases. There are few pathologists with both forensic and pediatric/perinatal expertise, and a dual doctor approach may be needed, but is expensive. The pathologist needs in these cases especially to be neutral, and ensure that both positive and negative findings are examined and documented as part of his examination, and the second part is making conclusions from the examination in the light of history, scans, previous tests, and ancillary investigations.

The forensic examination in some countries comes under a civil procedure, but in other countries, it is under the criminal law, and this can raise the stakes of any conclusions that are made on any clinical shortcomings that are identified. A medical approach can more readily investigate a mixture of system failings, and collate with other deaths and near misses.

Autopsy

The legal basis of the autopsy consists of several different categories by which a postmortem examination can occur, depending on the gestational age at birth (or sometimes the age at intrauterine demise), whether there were any signs of life (and how these are defined), and the legal position of the cause of death. These are discussed below.

Preregisterable Fetus

If the fetus is not registered (usually under 20/22/24/28 weeks according to jurisdiction), then apart from the exceptions above, these are usually medical examinations.

However, in many countries, the legal status of these bodies is not very clear. The legal state is like other surgical tissues and organ removed after a medical procedure, (from the mother—and the report usually goes into the mother's record) and many jurisdictions do not legally mandate consent for examination (i.e., similar to a placenta sent for examination), though the current expectations of society and ethical reviews require a formal consent process especially if incisions are to be made in the body of the fetus. It is interesting to note that fetal tissues are often regarded as special in many ethical reviews such as research use and somewhat different from other medical samples and tissues.

Registerable Fetus (Stillbirth)

In general to undertake a medical autopsy:

1. The medical certificate of fetal death/stillbirth should be completed in most jurisdictions.
2. Most jurisdictions would require a "maternal only" or parental consent.

3. Some jurisdictions require a human tissue act officer, or hospital medical director or nominated deputy to legally authorize the autopsy having sighted the parental consent.

There are some exceptions. Some jurisdictions (e.g., Qatar) allow a medical autopsy to be undertaken at the direction of the medical director if there is for an example an epidemic.

Consent can be an issue, one parent or both, and in some Muslim countries the father or next most senior male may feel he has the right. This needs careful consideration in the light of the social situation. However, there is growing support to the mother's rights in these areas, and ways to ensure her views are reflected are important.

The autopsy record may stay with the mother but often the stillbirth is given its own record number and medical file (whereas the placenta may go with mother or the fetus according to the hospital record procedure).

Mortuaries

Mortuaries usually need to be accredited to perform autopsies. In some jurisdictions, the site at which these can occur is also specifically mentioned by ministerial communication or law. In the UK, the human tissue authority provides guidelines on the facilities, and for example if emergency facilities are required.

Other rules and laws which may effect the operation of the mortuary are to do with prevention of infection, not allowing bodies to remain unrefrigerated, bodies and organs not to be retained for prolonged periods of time, and specific conditions such as body bags for infectious cases.

Religious Views on Postmortem and Burial

Religion in many countries influences the law, and also the ethical environment, so an appreciation of the religious views in the community one is working is important. In general there are some religious objections to the autopsy, and a natural human desire to prefer the body to "rest in peace, undisturbed" but most religions recognize the right of the country to investigate certain causes of death by law, and for people to have the right to have an autopsy to understand more why their relative died, or to help others through increasing knowledge [15]. There are several resources on the web to identify religious opinions on autopsy, and local religious leaders can also assist [16] and are very useful in creating guidelines.

Different religions have different ways of disposing of the body, by burial, cremation, or other means and not all countries will permit the range of options. In the Emirates, there are crematoria existing for Hindus and Christians, but in some other middle east countries cremation is not an option. Families who wish to cremate in these countries will need to go through repatriation, for cremation in their own country.

Organ Donation

This is not usually an issue for stillbirths, as tissue autolysis is too advanced, although the use of anencephalic neonates is under active discussion in some jurisdictions and occasional practice [17]. Some professional medical colleges have provided some thoughts on the use of anencephalic fetuses, and the UK donation ethics committee [18] and the AMA in the USA have provided cautious comments [19], but a Canadian paper has reached different conclusions [20]. The news headlines reporting these cases tend to focus on the altruism and benefit, and do not explore the ethical issues involved [21].

The mortuary though will be involved with these bodies after donation, and be aware that the body may go through surgery rather than straight from the ward although sometimes recovery of some tissues (corneas and heart valves) may be done in the mortuary if infection can be controlled. Different jurisdictions deal with organ donation differently, some an opt in (i.e., one has to consent or next of kin consent for donation to occur), others have an opt out where one is presumed to be a donor, unless opted out. The use of perinatal deaths for corneal donation and cardiac valves occurs [22].

The Medical Autopsy

This is usually to elucidate causes of death or obtain other information after a death certificate or similar has been completed. A forensic cause of death has therefore been excluded to the best of the ability of the clinician, and a reasonable cause of death has been ascertained as most likely or confirmed (though the error rate of death certificate is known to be quite high, and autopsy series in fetuses finds a different cause in 10–20% of cases). An autopsy may also uncover other important conditions only incidentally related to the death.

Some jurisdictions do not allow the medical autopsy, and others may place caveats. One is that the medical postmortem examination can occur, when the cause of death is unknown, but death is known to be due to natural causes. In this case it has to be unclear or unknown the exact process leading to the death although there are no suspicious features. This can require some care in the completion of the notification of death or the death certificate, for the autopsy to be legally permissible. For stillbirths, this is usually straightforward, as most are the result of a natural cause of death, albeit of unknown mechanism/mode. Other cases for example may be hydrops as the cause of death, but the cause of the hydrops is unknown.

The Forensic Autopsy

The forensic death will have as its focus more the determination as to whether there are legal issues with the death, negligence, trauma, and so on. This can mean that other findings, though of clinical interest, may not be of forensic interest. The forensic process separate from the hospital may also mean delays and a summary report provided to the hospital rather than a full autopsy report, depending on the jurisdiction. It may mean there is less feedback to the clinical areas, as this is peripheral to the function of the forensic examination. As there is usually no consent the process proceeds as the legal authorities see fit. Some jurisdictions may allow relatives to influence whether an autopsy forms part of the investigation [23].

Once the forensic investigation is completed, there are differing practices of retaining tissues and slides. Once the case is closed, the legal reasons for retaining them may cease, unless further legal actions are pending. In some cases, the process is to allow the return of slides and blocks to the family, which can preclude further review, especially if the process recurs in the family or further investigation is required. There may be a second consent process to enable retention and in the UK the main person to provide consent is identified by the Human Tissue Act, who may be a different person than the main contact of the forensic/coronial process [24].

An additional issue in some jurisdictions is the legal basis on which the investigation is carried out. In many western countries, it is under civil law and in the UK since the enactment of the Criminal Law Act 1977, coroners are no longer able to consider criminal liability as part of their investigations. The role of the coroner is to identify:

- Who the deceased was
- How, when, and where the deceased came by his or her death
- The particulars (if any) required for death to be registered concerning the death

In other countries, the public prosecutor who is undertaking the postmortem may be under criminal law and seeing whether persons are at fault. This may change the focus of the examination.

Consent Process

The medical autopsy requires consent in most jurisdictions, and ethically it is clear this is needed [25, 26]. This is often a legal requirement, though the process in several jurisdictions has changed from previous laws which were rather vague with "lack of objection" being a term used to permit an autopsy previously in the UK.

The consent process is a legal process and is not simple, for various factors. Who should sign? If the mother is not well should the father sign? If she is well and the culture is for the father to sign, how does the institution reflect her rights? Should both parents sign the consent? The processes dealing with these situations need to be discussed. The consent process needs to be tailored for the society as well as the law and the parents' state of mind, so the consent is meaningful despite their emotional stresses. The ability to take time to understand the process, and make a decision, and not under duress is important. Consent needs to be a process taken through with the parents, so their choice is informed and based not on their current feelings but how they may consider later when the questions of recurrence and cause are paramount. The use of bereavement councillors, information packs, and time to discuss with others including religious advisors is important.

As well as having an overview of the autopsy examination, the possibility of a limited, or minimally invasive and virtual autopsy may need to be covered. In many places, specific details of organ retention and how and if these are to be returned, the fact that slides and blocks are preferably to be kept for review, and the fact that ancillary investigations such as microbiological and genetic tests may have implications for the family need to be addressed. It also has to be recognized that although genetic disease investigations usually involve counselling, an autopsy may be to identify genetic diseases by morphological features alone (see below).

References

1. Freckelton I. Stillbirth and the law: options for law reform and issues for the coronial jurisdiction. J Law Med. 2013;21(1):7–26.
2. https://www.parliament.uk/documents/commons-library/Registration-of-stillbirth-SN05595.pdf.
3. https://www.rcog.org.uk/globalassets/documents/guidelines/goodpractice4registrationstillbirth2005.pdf.
4. Dickinson JE, Prime DK, Charles AK. The role of autopsy following pregnancy termination for fetal abnormality. Aust N Z J Obstet Gynaecol. 2007;47(6):445–9.
5. http://opac.oireachtas.ie/AWData/Library3/Bill_Digest_Health_Regulation_of_Termination_of_Pregnancy_Bill_131302.pdf.
6. Black KI, Douglas H, de Costa C. Women's access to abortion after 20 weeks' gestation for fetal chromosomal abnormalities: views and experiences of doctors in New South Wales and Queensland. Aust N Z J Obstet Gynaecol. 2015;55:144–8.
7. Sifris R, Belton S. Australia: abortion and human rights. Health Hum Rights. 2017; 19(1):209–20.
8. https://www.bma.org.uk/-/media/files/pdfs/employment%20advice/ethics/the-law-and-ethics-of-abortion-2018.pdf?la=en.
9. https://www.senat.fr/lc/lc280/lc280.pdf.
10. Gesser-Edelsburg A, NAE S. Decision-making on terminating pregnancy for Muslim Arab women pregnant with fetuses with congenital anomalies: maternal affect and doctor-patient communication. Reprod Health. 2017;14:49. https://doi.org/10.1186/s12978-017-0312-7.
11. Al-Matary A, Ali J. Controversies and considerations regarding the termination of pregnancy for Foetal Anomalies in Islam. BMC Med Ethics. 2014;15:10.
12. Collins K. Chapter 2 Neonaticide. In: Griest K, editor. Pediatric homicide medical investigation. Boca Raton: CRC Press Taylor & Francis; 2010. p. 25–38.
13. Byard RW. Sudden death in the young, chap. 13. 3rd ed. Cambridge: Cambridge University Press; 2010. p. 539–49.
14. Keeling JW. Chapter 10 Fetal and perinatal death. In: Busuttil A, Keeling J, editors. Paediatric and forensic medicine & pathology. London: Hodder Arnold; 2009. p. 180–97.
15. Gordijn SJ, Erwich JJ, Khong TY. The perinatal autopsy: pertinent issues in multicultural Western Europe. Eur J Obstet Gynecol Reprod Biol. 2007;132(1):3–7. Epub 2006 Nov 28.
16. https://emedicine.medscape.com/article/1705993-overview.
17. https://www.organdonation.nhs.uk/get-involved/news/our-baby-was-a-hero-parents-speak-one-year-on-from-their-baby-s-death/.
18. http://aomrc.org.uk/wp-content/uploads/2016/06/Organ_Donation_-infants_anencephaly_020316-2.pdf.
19. https://www.ama-assn.org/delivering-care/ethics/anencephalic-newborns-organ-donors.

20. Use of anencephalic newborns as organ donors. Paediatr Child Health. 2005;10(6):335–7.
21. https://www.bbc.com/ncws/hcalth-32425666.
22. http://carryingtoterm.org/donation-for-transplant-and-research.
23. https://www.coronerscourt.vic.gov.au/families/first-48-hours-families/forensic-process.
24. https://www.hta.gov.uk/policies/policy-consent-post-mortem-examination-and-tissue-reten-tion-under-human-tissue-act-2004.
25. https://www.hta.gov.uk/sites/default/files/Post-mortem_examination_-_your_choices_about_organs_and_tissue_FINAL_v3_0_0.pdf.
26. http://www.health.wa.gov.au/postmortem/.

Consent for Medical Autopsy

Adrian Charles

In many countries as well as the consent as above, legally the autopsy is authorized by a human tissue act officer or medical director or their nominee, who legally allows the postmortem to go ahead. This is done after maternal or parental consent. Consent is now recognised to be a process, a communication and understanding, and not just a simple signature to an official form [1].

In Muslim countries, there may be comments in the law that a female doctor performs the autopsy on a female, if available (particularly for postpubertal females).

Genetic Testing

Consent in these cases may be a two-step process, tissue retained at autopsy for genetic analysis (if necessary with parental samples—trio testing) after consent for DNA confirmation is obtained at postmortem follow-up. This is an area that should be discussed with the fetal medicine and geneticists so a clear process occurs, for the local laws and ethical principles.

There are now a number of guidelines on genetic testing [2–4]. However, still-births do create some challenges. At autopsy there are many conditions where the morphology may give a definite genetic diagnosis, without DNA testing, yet specific consent for genetic testing has not been obtained. Though, this is also true in other clinical situations in the outpatient clinic or ward. However, the test sample needs to be taken. It can therefore be helpful to comply with laws and guides that specific consent for genetic diagnosis is needed, that the postmortem consent or information leaflet can explain that sometimes a genetic disease may be identified (which may not be related to the fetal loss) and this will be discussed later (usually

A. Charles (✉)
Anatomical Pathology, Sidra Medicine, Doha, Qatar

Clinical Pathology and Laboratory Medicine, Weil Cornell College of Medicine, Doha, Qatar
e-mail: acharles@sidra.org

© Springer Nature Switzerland AG 2021
J. Martinovic (ed.), *Practical Manual of Fetal Pathology*,
https://doi.org/10.1007/978-3-030-42492-3_3

before genetic confirmation). Even this is not always straightforward, as the pathologist may have a differential diagnosis, and to complete the autopsy report needs the genetic test for confirmation, or excluding various conditions. These scenarios require a close working relationship between the fetal medicine staff, clinical genetics staff, and the parents. It can be difficult when one has got features which could be a recurrent disease, but may not be, to issue a report with caveats, when a genetic test can be definitive. For example a fetus with some soft signs suggestive of, but may well not be trisomy 21 can be easily excluded, rather than issuing a report raising the possibility of Trisomy 21 which can mislead. A test confirming either way means a clearer report. This can be clarified in the consent or information sheet as to the extent of routine fetal genetic tests that may be done, such as routine fetal chromosomal array.

Other genetic issues arising from this area are paternity testing and the use of stored neonatal screening cards for legal or criminal identification purposes (including the parents), which has caused concerns [5].

Infectious Disease

The mortuary is a place that is under close inspection by regulatory agencies for control on infectious disease, with rules on the use of body bags and when and what precautions are required. Another ethical and possibly legal issue can be the routine testing of bodies undertaken in some mortuaries for blood borne infectious disease, prior to autopsy, as this is indirectly testing the mother without her consent.

Retention and Disposal of Tissues and Organs

Many pathology credentialing organizations (e.g., CAP, NEQAS) require tissues taken for diagnosis to be kept for review. This can conflict with parental wishes for all tissues to be returned. Virtual microscopy can assist in this. The benefits of long-term storage for review need to be explained in the information sheet.

Organs, and particularly the heart and the brain, may well need specific consent for retention (and is good practice), unless rapid process allows the examination to take place at the same time.

The placenta can also be an organ that is regarded as precious and required to be returned to the mother by some societies, such as the Maori [6].

The status of the post morten and fetal tissues, under whose ownership, and what uses they can be used for are legal and ethical questions that differ in different societies.

Research

Embryonic tissues are not really part of this topic, but research on human embryonic tissue is strictly regulated, especially stem cell research, and it has been a focus of much debate with opposing views.

Fetal tissues are usually allowed to be involved in research, but even the previable fetal tissues are usually regarded as special and not the same as "routine surgical pathology" tissues as mentioned above. A demonstration of the change in time of ethical concensus is the Polkinghorne report in the UK in 1989 suggested fetal research was permissible, but suggested the specifics of the research was not needed, which has since been superseded by the Human Tissue Act requiring more specific informed consent.

Genetic research is another difficult topic. Consent is needed for research and this may be specific, or retained as part of a more general biobank according to the ethics and laws. A more nuanced consent process may be the way forward [7].

Public Display

Body Worlds and Gunther von Hagens demonstrations of the human anatomy have created various reactions. Although Museum collections of fetuses and organs from autopsy around the world in hospital and university museums have in the past been collected according to old ethical standards, some of these collections have been disposed of, but still today there is much value in these collections. It is important to review what laws apply to collections held, and especially in public areas, that correct consent is covered or appropriately "grandfathered" in recognizing that ethical values change, and old consent procedures may not reflect today's value, but the loss of irreplaceable material requires a balanced approach. In the UK, such exhibitions need to be licensed. In France in 2009 the Body works exhibition was closed for commercializing the body but also with questions raised on the provenance of the bodies [8].

Disposal of Bodies

Usually bodies are disposed to the family or the funeral director for burial or cremation, though repatriation may occur in an expatriate setting. Some jurisdictions have limits on how long a body can be stored in a healthcare facility and processes to deal with these situations need to be addressed. Occasional abandoned bodies can cause issues with no family to contact and will require careful disposal with involvement of the hospital executive and local authorities.

Burial and Cremation

Disposal of the preregistered babies in the UK has some guidelines [9]. Other jurisdictions have varying guidelines. In some jurisdictions, the cemetery legally requires
a certificate to be able to bury these cases, especially individual burials. For previable fetuses, some jurisdictions allow group burials. Muslim remains should be buried no matter the gestational age (previable fetuses as a group and also
largelimb amputation surgical specimens) in specified permitted areas. Burial usually takes place for Muslims within a day or so of death.

Cremation is preferred by the Hindu, but not acceptable to Muslims. Some
Muslim countries (e.g., Emirates) provide a cremation service for certain religious
groups. Other jurisdictions allow arrangements with crematoria, or the hospital having a dedicated cremation facility with permission for these cases (though usually
limited to previable fetuses/stillbirths, organs, and amputations) [10].

Burial sites tend to be religiously segregated, and in many Muslim countries
there are special graveyards for non-Muslims. For some countries, there is a legal
paper to allow the body to be buried that needs to be obtained after completing the
legal formalities.

Many countries have rules on where the burial can occur and where ashes can be
scattered.

Repatriation is a common occurrence in the Middle East, including occasionally
stillbirth. This has to comply with local laws, the laws of the country being returned
and rules on air freight.

Privacy Laws After Death

Though the health information after death has often not been respected, privacy
guidelines from the United States (HIPAA) have clear guidelines, and there is a 50
year rule following the death protecting a deceased person's identifiable health
information [11].

Further privacy-related issues can come about from where the medical record of
the baby is kept—in its own record, or the mother's record and where the placental
report is kept. If the father wants a copy, is any medical information related to the
mother in the stillbirth history that may be an issue?

New Moves

There have been legal arguments (see ref [12]) and discussions at governmental
level in several countries (e.g., Australia [13], and the UK [14]) for the coronial
system take over the investigation of Stillbirths. This has arisen from patchy access
to good postmortem examinations and in general the variable investigations of stillbirths. Australia is now considering funding for postmortem examinations in these
cases through medicare to increase the availability of this investigation.

The mandatory coronial investigation has merit, in ensuring investigation of all cases, but the number of stillbirths (around 5 for every 1000 live births) and the expertise required from a multidisciplinary team who will not normally be working in a legal framework, ensuring quick and timely reports and open discussion in a legal setting may be difficult and expensive. The mandatory coronial approach also removes the current choice the parents have for postmortem examination. A paternalistic attitude has caused big problems in the past, and money may be better spent on developing regional centers of excellence with a strong parental input.

The other area that has increasing pressure is the human rights that a fetus has. This has been driven partly by antiabortion activists in the USA, but also is at the heart of the ethical decision of when is a human a human, and when in development does this occur, when even birth is a process and not a single point of transition. This will again affect the laws around postmortem and the tissues, and the information from genetic studies in these cases.

Final Considerations

The autopsy remains an important way to answer questions of why a baby died. It has considerable value to provide answers to the parents, and the wider family with certain genetic diseases. The information from the autopsy is also helpful to medical practice and the hospital, and data is used for government statistics and registries. The stillbirth rate provides a key indicator of healthcare of a community. There have been several important recent initiatives such as the recent Lancet reviews (2011 and 2016 see below), the CDC in the USA, and the combined parental and professional interest groups (e.g., International Stillbirth Alliance [12]) to focus on reducing stillbirths. However, it is a sensitive area and laws and ethical practices need to be carefully reviewed and policies and procedures implemented.

This review is not meant to be comprehensive, but indicates areas where someone setting up or running a fetal autopsy service should ascertain what laws and guidelines are pertinent and sensitive to the country and state they practice, and also the culture and religious practices and thoughts of the people whom they serve. When running a service it is important to be aware of these issues, and constantly review the practice to see standards are being maintained, laws (and new ones) pertinent to the area are addressed, and the cultures of the families dealing with the mortuary are being respected. This may require translators and people familiar with these customs to advise. It is important to maintain discussions with the bereaved to reduce the risk of further inquiries.

Checklists: A Guide!

Check with the laws covering registering births and stillbirths and autopsies to see what is covered, the ages that apply, and the reasons to investigate.

Special regulations around fetal tissue and gonadal tissue.

Consider having a similar pathway for recognizable human fetal remains of all gestational ages, and although a legal authorization is needed for examination for a registered birth, a similar consent procedure should be used for invasive examinations under this gestational age.

Good practice and ethics indicate that consent is required for all non legal/forensic fetal invasive autopsies. For an external review only this may be more informal as in a well-baby check on a live baby.

Check local religious leaders, for their opinions.

Aim to comply with ethical best practice, which may be more stringent than the law, particularly if the laws are old or not very clear.

Know the communities one is working with, their faiths and views, but every couple is different ad processes should be flexible to be lawful and ethical but also respond to parental wishes. There may need to be nuanced approach—with a range of services offered (some Muslim and Jewish babies may be requested to be examined and buried quickly and once shrouded not disturbed).

Sensitive approach to the autopsy—keep incisions as small as reasonable and neat, reconstruct, return as much of the organs as reasonably possible.

Develop consent forms and parent information packs.

Get a bereavement team who can form a point of contact for the parents after they leave the hospital.

Work with parent groups (e.g., Sids and Kids, Sands, etc.); the hospital and practice must conform to in with society norms and keep moving as society changes.

Adopt and develop new processes and approach to autopsy including virtual autopsy with MRI, CT, and ultrasound postmortem scans, and minimally invasive procedures.

Be available to see parents before autopsy and after at the follow-up clinic.

References

1. http://www.health.wa.gov.au/postmortem/docs/Non-Coronial_Post-Mortem_Examinations_Code_of_Practice_2007.pdf.
2. http://www.eurogentest.org/index.php?id=732.
3. https://ghr.nlm.nih.gov/primer/testing/informedconsent/.
4. Clayton EW, Evans BJ, Hazel JW, Rothstein MA. The law of genetic privacy: applications, implications, and limitations. J Law Biosci. 2019;6(1):1–36.
5. Bowman DM, Studdert DM. Newborn screening cards: a legal quagmire. Med J Aust. 2011;194(6):319–22.
6. https://www.hauoratairawhiti.org.nz/assets/Uploads/Perinatal-Post-Mortem-and-Placenta-Histopathology.pdf.
7. Panikkar B, Smith N, Brown P. Reflexive research ethics in fetal tissue xenotransplantation research. Account Res. 2012;19(6):344–69. https://doi.org/10.1080/08989621.2012.728910.
8. https://www.france24.com/en/20100917-our-body-controversial-exhibition-france-appeal-court-ban-china-prisons-justice-arts.

9. https://www.hta.gov.uk/sites/default/files/Guidance_on_the_disposal_of_pregnancy_
    remains.pdf.
10. https://www.parliament.wa.gov.au/publications/tabledpapers.nsf/displaypaper/401028
    7c460594b047609650482581460003fbc2/$file/tp-287.pdf.
11. https://www.hhs.gov/hipaa/for-professionals/privacy/guidance/health-information-of-
    deceased-individuals/index.html.
12. https://stillbirthalliance.org.
13. https://www.aph.gov.au/Parliamentary_Business/Committees/Senate/Stillbirth_Research_
    and_Education/Stillbirth. Accessed 2/11/2019.
14. https://www.gov.uk/government/news/new-powers-to-investigate-stillbirths. Accessed 2/11/2019.

Further Reading[1]

Australia has sets of guidelines and rules covering mortuary and associated facilities. https://
    aushfg-prod-com-au.s3.amazonaws.com/HPU_B.0490_6_0.pdf. Some states have local gov-
    ernment acts that control these. https://www.health.nsw.gov.au/environment/dotd/Documents/
    disposal-of-bodies-ph-reg-2012.pdf.
BMA. Medical ethics today, chap. 12. In: Medical ethics today: the BMA's handbook of ethics and
    law hardcover. 3rd ed. Wiley; 2012.
http://www.health.wa.gov.au/postmortem/docs/Non-Coronial_Post-Mortem_Examinations_
    Code_of_Practice_2007.pdf.
https://www.legislation.wa.gov.au/legislation/statutes.nsf/law_s40132.html.
https://sanda.psanz.com.au/clinical-practice/clinical-guidelines/.
https://sanda.psanz.com.au/assets/Uploads/Section-4-PerintalPostMortemExaminatio
    n-V3-100418.pdf.
International Stillbirth Alliance. https://stillbirthalliance.org.
March of dimes. https://www.marchofdimes.org/complications/stillbirth.aspx.
Mortuary references. https://www.hta.gov.uk/policies/policy-consent-post-mortem-examination-
    and-tissue-retention-under-human-tissue-act-2004.
Review on religions Medscape. https://emedicine.medscape.com/article/1705993-overview#a1.
The two Lancet series: 2011. https://www.thelancet.com/series/stillbirth; 2016. https://www.thel-
    ancet.com/series/ending-preventable-stillbirths.
The World Health Organisation. https://www.who.int/maternal_child_adolescent/topics/maternal/
    maternal_perinatal/en/.
USA Center for Disease Control. https://www.cdc.gov/ncbddd/stillbirth/index.html.

---

[1] The following publications and websites may offer helpful information.

Part II

Fetal Biometry

Abstract

Taking and recording measurements and organ weights has always been an essential point in postmortem examinations generating series of good charts through the history, many of these still widely used. Fetal measurements taken as a part of routine ultrasound scan examinations—dating, anomaly, and growth scan—provide valuable resource of data for the perinatal pathologist. Measurements taken during the autopsy often reflect multiple artifactual changes, making their interpretation complex and sometimes challenging, but remaining an essential diagnostic tool, especially when carefully correlated with the clinical history and with other pathological findings. True and significant anomalies of fetal and neonatal measurements can indicate maternal disease, underlying genetic condition, congenital malformations, environmental or socioeconomic problems. In this chapter, we aim to briefly introduce the widely used postmortem measurement techniques and discuss possible artifacts, while keeping in focus the interpretation of postmortem data in context of fetal growth problems.

Body Measurements

Beata Hargitai

All measurement has to be compared with and assessed against the "normal" value for the length of gestation. Determination of gestational age and minimum set of data, required for postmortem report, will be discussed in this paragraph.

Obstetric Ultrasonographic Fetal Biometry

Gestational age is usually calculated by weeks (or weeks plus days) and the base of calculation is the time of the last menstrual period (LMP) which is refined by results of the "dating ultrasound scan," as recollection of dates by the gravida is not always reliable. The dating scan is ideally performed in the first trimester, between 11 and 13+6/40 weeks of gestation, or earlier, to determine gestational age based on fetal measurements—traditionally CRL (crown-rump length) and BPD (biparietal diameter)—and to establish the expected date of delivery. Instead of BPD, head circumference (occipito-frontal circumference, OFC) appears to be more accurate, to follow up fetal growth and to estimate fetal size later in gestation head circumference, abdominal circumference, and femur length are the recommended tools [1, 2] (Tables 1, 2, 3).

Large discrepancy between gestational age "by dates" and "by scan" can indicate profound problem of fetal growth in viable fetus and may help to determine length of in utero retention following intrauterine fetal death.

B. Hargitai (✉)
West Midlands Perinatal Pathology, Birmingham Women's and Children's Hospital, Birmingham, UK
e-mail: Beata.Hargitai@nhs.net

© Springer Nature Switzerland AG 2021
J. Martinovic (ed.), *Practical Manual of Fetal Pathology*,
https://doi.org/10.1007/978-3-030-42492-3_4

Table 1 Ultrasonographic crown-rump length dating table (5–14 weeks of gestation)

CRL (mm)	GA (weeks + days)		
	50th centile	5th centile	95th centile
5	6 + 0	5 + 2	6 + 5
6	6 + 2	5 + 4	7 + 0
7	6 + 3	5 + 6	7 + 1
8	6 + 5	6 + 0	7 + 2
9	6 + 6	6 + 2	7 + 4
10	7 + 1	6 + 3	7 + 5
11	7 + 2	6 + 4	8 + 0
12	7 + 3	6 + 5	8 + 1
13	7 + 4	7 + 0	8 + 2
14	7 + 5	7 + 1	8 + 3
15	7 + 6	7 + 2	8 + 4
16	8 + 1	7 + 3	8 + 5
17	8 + 2	7 + 4	8 + 6
18	8 + 3	7 + 5	9 + 0
19	8 + 3	7 + 6	9 + 1
20	8 + 4	8 + 0	9 + 2
21	8 + 5	8 + 1	9 + 3
22	8 + 6	8 + 1	9 + 4
23	9 + 0	8 + 2	9 + 5
24	9 + 1	8 + 3	9 + 6
25	9 + 2	8 + 4	9 + 6
26	9 + 3	8 + 5	10 + 0
27	9 + 3	8 + 6	10 + 1
28	9 + 4	8 + 6	10 + 2
29	9 + 5	9 + 0	10 + 3
30	9 + 6	9 + 1	10 + 3
31	9 + 6	9 + 2	10 + 4
32	10 + 0	9 + 2	10 + 5
33	10 + 1	9 + 3	10 + 6
34	10 + 2	9 + 4	10 + 6
35	10 + 2	9 + 5	11 + 0
36	10 + 3	9 + 5	11 + 1
37	10 + 4	9 + 6	11 + 1
38	10 + 4	10 + 0	11 + 2
39	10 + 5	10 + 0	11 + 3
40	10 + 6	10 + 1	11 + 3
41	10 + 6	10 + 2	11 + 4
42	11 + 0	10 + 2	11 + 5
43	11 + 0	10 + 3	11 + 5
44	11 + 1	10 + 3	11 + 6
45	11 + 2	10 + 4	11 + 6
46	11 + 2	10 + 5	12 + 0
47	11 + 3	10 + 5	12 + 1
48	11 + 4	10 + 6	12 + 1

Table 1 (continued)

CRL (mm)	GA (weeks + days)		
	50th centile	5th centile	95th centile
49	11 + 4	10 + 6	12 + 2
50	11 + 5	11 + 0	12 + 2
51	11 + 5	11 + 1	12 + 3
52	11 + 6	11 + 1	12 + 4
53	11 + 6	11 + 2	12 + 4
54	12 + 0	11 + 2	12 + 5
55	12 + 1	11 + 3	12 + 5
56	12 + 1	11 + 3	12 + 6
57	12 + 2	11 + 4	12 + 6
58	12 + 2	11 + 4	13 + 0
59	12 + 3	11 + 5	13 + 0
60	12 + 3	11 + 6	13 + 1
61	12 + 4	11 + 6	13 + 1
62	12 + 4	12 + 0	13 + 2
63	12 + 5	12 + 0	13 + 3
64	12 + 5	12 + 1	13 + 3
65	12 + 6	12 + 1	13 + 4
66	12 + 6	12 + 2	13 + 4
67	13 + 0	12 + 2	13 + 5
68	13 + 0	12 + 3	13 + 5
69	13 + 1	12 + 3	13 + 6
70	13 + 1	12 + 4	13 + 6
71	13 + 2	12 + 4	14 + 0
72	13 + 2	12 + 5	14 + 0
73	13 + 3	12 + 5	14 + 0
74	13 + 3	12 + 6	14 + 1
75	13 + 4	12 + 6	14 + 1
76	13 + 4	13 + 0	14 + 2
77	13 + 5	13 + 0	14 + 2
78	13 + 5	13 + 0	14 + 3
79	13 + 6	13 + 1	14 + 3
80	13 + 6	13 + 1	14 + 4

From Ultrasound 2009;17(3):161–167 Fetal size and dating: charts recommended for clinical obstetric practice. Pam Loughna, Lyn Chitty, Tony Evans, and Trish Chudleigh with permissions

Charts recommended for clinical obstetric practice for the estimation and follow-up of fetal growth have been published and revisited by large national and international organizations [3–8]. Fetal biometry based on ultrasonography is essential tool in clinical diagnosis of fetal growth anomalies and can be helpful in perinatal pathology as well—from first trimester to term—when examining non-macerated fetuses.

Table 2 Ultrasonographic head circumference dating table (11–39 weeks of gestation)

Head circumference (mm)	GA (weeks + days)		
	50th centile	5th centile	95th centile
80	12 + 4	11 + 3	13 + 5
85	12 + 6	11 + 6	14 + 1
90	13 + 2	12 + 2	14 + 4
95	13 + 5	12 + 4	15 + 0
100	14 + 1	13 + 0	15 + 3
105	14 + 4	13 + 3	15 + 5
110	15 + 0	13 + 6	16 + 1
115	15 + 3	14 + 2	16 + 4
120	15 + 6	14 + 5	17 + 0
125	16 + 2	15 + 1	17 + 3
130	16 + 4	15 + 4	17 + 6
135	17 + 0	15 + 6	18 + 2
140	17 + 3	16 + 2	18 + 5
145	17 + 6	16 + 5	19 + 1
150	18 + 2	17 + 1	19 + 3
155	18 + 5	17 + 4	19 + 6
160	19 + 1	17 + 6	20 + 2
165	19 + 3	18 + 2	20 + 5
170	19 + 6	18 + 5	21 + 1
175	20 + 2	19 + 1	21 + 4
180	20 + 5	19 + 3	22 + 0
185	21 + 1	19 + 6	22 + 3
190	21 + 4	20 + 2	22 + 6
195	22 + 0	20 + 4	23 + 2
200	22 + 2	21 + 0	23 + 5
205	22 + 5	21 + 3	24 + 2
210	23 + 1	21 + 5	24 + 5
215	23 + 4	22 + 1	25 + 1
220	24 + 0	22 + 4	25 + 5
225	24 + 3	22 + 6	26 + 1
230	24 + 6	23 + 2	26 + 5
235	25 + 3	23 + 5	27 + 1
240	25 + 6	24 + 1	27 + 5
245	26 + 2	24 + 3	28 + 2
250	26 + 5	24 + 6	28 + 6
255	27 + 2	25 + 2	29 + 3
260	27 + 5	25 + 5	30 + 0
265	28 + 2	26 + 1	30 + 4
270	28 + 6	26 + 4	31 + 2
275	29 + 3	27 + 0	32 + 0
280	30 + 0	27 + 3	32 + 4
285	30 + 4	27 + 6	33 + 3
290	31 + 1	28 + 3	34 + 1

Table 2 (continued)

Head circumference (mm)	GA (weeks + days)		
	50th centile	5th centile	95th centile
295	31 + 5	28 + 6	35 + 0
300	32 + 3	29 + 3	35 + 6
305	33 + 1	30 + 0	36 + 5
310	33 + 6	30 + 3	37 + 4
315	34 + 4	31 + 0	38 + 4
320	35 + 3	31 + 5	39 + 4

From Ultrasound 2009;17(3):161–167 Fetal size and dating: charts recommended for clinical obstetric practice. Pam Loughna, Lyn Chitty, Tony Evans, and Trish Chudleigh with permissions

Table 3 Ultrasonographic femur length dating table (12–38 weeks of gestation)

Femur length (mm)	GA (weeks + days)		
	50th centile	5th centile	95th centile
10	13 + 0	12 + 1	13 + 6
11	13 + 2	12 + 3	14 + 1
12	13 + 4	12 + 5	14 + 4
13	13 + 6	13 + 0	14 + 6
14	14 + 1	13 + 1	15 + 1
15	14 + 3	13 + 3	15 + 3
16	14 + 5	13 + 5	15 + 6
17	15 + 0	14 + 0	16 + 1
18	15 + 2	14 + 2	16 + 3
19	15 + 5	14 + 4	16 + 6
20	16 + 0	14 + 6	17 + 1
21	16 + 2	15 + 1	17 + 3
22	16 + 4	15 + 3	17 + 6
23	16 + 6	15 + 5	18 + 1
24	17 + 2	16 + 0	18 + 4
25	17 + 4	16 + 2	18 + 6
26	17 + 6	16 + 4	19 + 2
27	18 + 2	16 + 6	19 + 5
28	18 + 4	17 + 1	20 + 0
29	18 + 6	17 + 4	20 + 3
30	19 + 2	17 + 6	20 + 5
31	19 + 4	18 + 1	21 + 1
32	20 + 0	18 + 3	21 + 4
33	20 + 2	18 + 5	22 + 0
34	20 + 5	19 + 1	22 + 2
35	21 + 0	19 + 3	22 + 5
36	21 + 3	19 + 5	23 + 1
37	21 + 5	20 + 1	32 + 4
38	22 + 1	20 + 3	24 + 0

(continued)

Table 3 (continued)

Femur length (mm)	GA (weeks + days)		
	50th centile	5th centile	95th centile
39	22 + 4	20 + 5	24 + 3
40	22 + 6	21 + 1	24 + 6
41	23 + 2	21 + 3	25 + 2
42	23 + 5	21 + 6	25 + 5
43	24 + 1	22 + 1	26 + 1
44	24 + 3	22 + 4	26 + 4
45	24 + 6	22 + 6	27 + 1
46	25 + 2	23 + 2	27 + 4
47	25 + 5	23 + 4	28 + 0
48	26 + 1	24 + 0	28 + 3
49	26 + 4	24 + 3	29 + 0
50	27 + 0	24 + 5	29 + 3
51	27 + 3	25 + 1	30 + 0
52	27 + 6	25 + 4	30 + 3
53	28 + 2	26 + 0	31 + 0
54	28 + 5	26 + 2	31 + 3
55	29 + 2	26 + 5	32 + 0
56	29 + 5	27 + 1	32 + 3
57	30 + 1	27 + 4	33 + 0
58	30 + 4	28 + 0	33 + 4
59	31 + 1	28 + 3	34 + 1
60	31 + 4	28 + 6	34 + 4
61	32 + 1	29 + 2	35 + 1
62	32 + 4	29 + 5	35 + 5
63	33 + 1	30 + 1	36 + 2
64	33 + 4	30 + 4	36 + 6
65	34 + 1	31 + 0	37 + 3
66	34 + 4	31 + 3	38 + 0
67	35 + 1	32 + 0	38 + 5

From Ultrasound 2009;17(3):161–167 Fetal size and dating: charts recommended for clinical obstetric practice. Pam Loughna, Lyn Chitty, Tony Evans, and Trish Chudleigh with permissions

Pathological Fetal Biometry: Minimum Dataset

Thorough and meticulous measurement and recording of growth parameters is an essential part of the perinatal postmortem examination [9–13]. The technique of using the ruler, a piece of string, and calipers is not complicated but needs appropriate training. A good quality, regularly serviced scale is necessary to obtain reliable organ measurements. Measuring babies with developmental anomalies i.e., skeletal, vertebral malformations or severely macerated bodies with lax joints and formalin fixed cases may require different approach and practical experience. Measurements can be taken using digital images, i.e., long bones can be measured on postmortem radiology images. It is a good practice to record the collected measurements not only at the beginning of the postmortem report but feeding into a database which later can be used to create institutional population based statistics.

Systematic biometric linear measurements are essential parts of the minimum dataset and include body length (crown heel length, CHL, distance of the vertex of calvarium and the sole), sitting length (crown-rump length, CRL, measured from the vertex to the most distant point of the buttock), foot length (toe-heel length, measured between the posterior prominence of the calcaneus and the tip of the longest toe), head circumference (occipito-frontal circumference, OFC, measured above the eyebrows anteriorly and the most distant point of the occiput posteriorly). OFC and CR length tend to equal as do femur length and foot length. Linear measurements are measured in cm, round to tenth or in mm. Chest circumference (CCF, measured in the transverse plain at the level of nipples), and abdominal circumference (ACF, measured at the level of umbilicus) albeit widely used in obstetric practice on ultrasound assessment, can be biased by the degree of postmortem changes and are not helpful in macerated cases (Fig. 1a–d). Standardization by

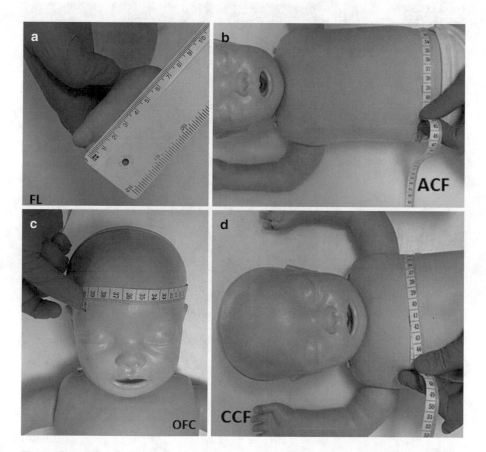

Fig. 1 Technique of taking fetal postmortem external body measurements (**a**) (*FL* foot length, (**b**) *ACF* abdominal circumference, (**c**) *OFC* occipito-frontal circumference or head circumference, (**d**) *CCF* chest circumference)

anthropometry can help to identify growth problems, developmental abnormalities, major facial anomalies, and minor dysmorphic features, thus providing valuable input for the clinical geneticists. Inner and outer canthal distances (distance between the inner canthi and outer canthi of the eyes), eye fissure length, interpupillary distance (distance between the centers of pupils or midpoints of eyelids), philtrum length (distance between the external end of nasal septum and the midline depression of the upper lip), inter-nipple distance (measurement between the midpoints of the nipples), and hand length are frequently used parameters in genetic autopsies [13–16] (Fig. 2).

Measurements can be taken for all long bones on postmortem X-ray if necessary. Standard curves of long bone measurements for comparison however are based on ultrasound scan measurements.

In addition to linear measurements, body weight and organ weights have essential role in the postmortem report. The body has to be weighed without wrapping,

Fig. 2 Facial measurements. *IPD* interpupillary distance, *ICD* intercanthal distance, *OCD* outer canthal distance, *PL* philtrum length

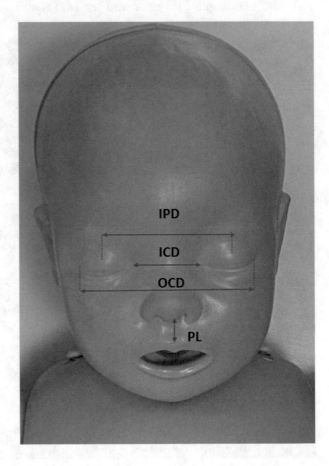

clothes, and with cannula removed. Whenever possible, customized body weight (birth weight) centile has to be calculated. Body weight measurement is given to the postmortem report in grams as are the organ weights, round to the nearest tenth. Deviation from normal values should be quantified by SD or percentile. Centiles over 90% and below 10% and deviation of more than 1 SD are conventionally considered as abnormal.

Examination of the placenta is part of the perinatal postmortem, and weight and measurements have to be taken and recorded similarly to biometrical parameters of the infant. Examination of the placenta is discussed and standard tables are recommended in separate chapter "Examination of the Placenta."

Use of standard birth weight, organ weight and linear measurement tables and curves, and principles of choosing reference charts are discussed in the following subsection.

Pathological Determination of Gestational Age

In autopsy cases of recent perinatal death, fresh stillbirth, or spontaneous miscarriage, if referred with an accurately (by scan) and timely (first trimester) determined gestational age, fetal measurements and organ weights can be compared to the respective figures of postmortem measurement charts directly.

In case of non-macerated fetuses with indeterminate gestational age—in setting of un-booked or concealed pregnancies—foot length, below 29 weeks, and considering individual variations afterwards; and femur length, measured on postmortem X-ray, are reliable indicators of gestational age. In addition, other morphological indicators and milestones of development and organ maturation—from gyral pattern of the brain to appearance of various ossification centers, radial alveolar count, skin or renal cortical development—can aid with the determination of fetal age and these are discussed in detail in the chapter "Fetal Autopsy."

In a severely macerated fetus pathological assessment of the gestational age albeit necessary, is often challenging—e.g., myelination pattern of the central nervous system, number of generations of glomeruli in the renal cortex, or other fine histological maturation markers provide scarce information. Examiners often experience that CRL, CHL, and especially OFC measurements are affected by maceration, and therefore of little use in severely macerated cases, while foot length can still help to determine gestational age—except when feet are dried out and mummified. Accurately measured femur length can be very helpful if postmortem X-ray is available. Taking femur measurement on babygram is a straightforward technique (Fig. 3).

Table 4 aids postmortem dating based on radiological measurement of the femur.

Fig. 3 Taking femur
length measurement on
computer
radiography imager

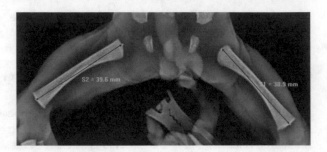

Table 4 Femur length dating table (11–42 weeks of gestation postmortem X-ray, BWC Hospital Data)

Gestational week biometry	("Femur (mm)," "3rd percentile")	("Femur (mm)," "10th percentile")	("Femur (mm)," "50th percentile")	("Femur (mm)," "90th percentile")	("Femur (mm)," "97th percentile")
11	4	4	6	8	10
12	4	4	8	10	12
13	8	8	12	12	14
14	10	12	14	16	16
15	12	14	16	20	20
16	16	16	20	22	24
17	16	20	22	24	26
18	20	24	24	28	28
19	24	24	28	32	32
20	26	28	32	34	36
21	28	32	34	36	38
22	32	32	36	40	40
23	34	36	40	42	44
24	36	36	40	44	44
25	34	38	44	48	48
26	38	42	46	48	52
27	40	44	48	52	52
28	44	46	52	54	56
29	42	48	52	56	58
30	48	48	56	60	62
31	52	52	58	64	64
32	52	56	60	64	66
33	58	60	64	66	68
34	60	60	64	68	70
35	60	64	68	72	72
36	64	64	68	72	76
37	64	66	72	76	78
38	66	68	72	78	80

Table 4 (continued)

Gestational week biometry	("Femur (mm)," "3rd percentile")	("Femur (mm)," "10th percentile")	("Femur (mm)," "50th percentile")	("Femur (mm)," "90th percentile")	("Femur (mm)," "97th percentile")
39	66	70	76	80	82
40	70	72	78	80	84
41	74	76	80	84	84
42	76	76	80	82	84

References

1. Loughna P, Chitty L, Evans T, Chudleigh T. Fetal size and dating: charts recommended for clinical obstetric practice. Ultrasound. 2009;17(3):161–7. https://doi.org/10.117 9/174313409X448543.
2. Butt K, Lim K, Diagnostic Imaging Committee. Determination of gestational age by ultrasound. J Obstet Gynaecol Can. 2014;36(2):171–81. https://doi.org/10.1016/S1701-2163(15)30664-2.
3. Kiserud T, Benachi A, Hecher K, Perez RG, Carvalho J, Piaggio G, Platt LD. The World Health Organization fetal growth charts: concept, findings, interpretation, and application. Am J Obstet Gynecol. 2018;218(2S):S619–29. https://doi.org/10.1016/j.ajog.2017.12.010.
4. Villar J, Cheikh Ismail L, Victora CG, Ohuma EO, Bertino E, Altman DG, Lambert A, Papageorghiou AT, Carvalho M, Jaffer YA, Gravett MG, Purwar M, Frederick IO, Noble AJ, Pang R, Barros FC, Chumlea C, Bhutta ZA, Kennedy SH, International Fetal and Newborn Growth Consortium for the 21st Century (INTERGROWTH-21st). International standards for newborn weight, length, and head circumference by gestational age and sex: the Newborn Cross-Sectional Study of the INTERGROWTH-21st Project. Lancet. 2014;384(9946):857–68. https://doi.org/10.1016/S0140-6736(14)60932-6.
5. Salomon LJ, Alfirevic Z, Da Silva CF, Deter RL, Figueras F, Ghi T, Glanc P, Khalil A, Lee W, Napolitano R, Papageorghiou A, Sotiriadis A, Stirnemann J, Toi A, Yeo G. ISUOG practice guidelines: ultrasound assessment of fetal biometry and growth. Ultrasound Obstet Gynecol. 2019;53(6):715–23. https://doi.org/10.1002/uog.20272.
6. Vayssière C, Sentilhes L, Ego A, Bernard C, Cambourieu D, Flamant C, Gascoin G, Gaudineau A, Grangé G, Houfflin-Debarge V, Langer B, Malan V, Marcorelles P, Nizard J, Perrotin F, Salomon L, Senat MV, Serry A, Tessier V, Truffert P, Tsatsaris V, Arnaud C, Carbonne B. Fetal growth restriction and intra-uterine growth restriction: guidelines for clinical practice from the French College of Gynaecologists and Obstetricians. Eur J Obstet Gynecol Reprod Biol. 2015;193:10–8. https://doi.org/10.1016/j.ejogrb.2015.06.021. Epub 2015 Jul 2.
7. Wigglesworth JS, Singer DB, editors. Textbook of fetal and perinatal pathology, vol. 2. 2nd ed. Malden: Blackwell Science; 1998.
8. Khong TY. The perinatal necropsy. In: Khong TY, Malcomson RDG, editors. Keeling's fetal and neonatal pathology. 5th ed. London: Springer; 2015.
9. Gilbert-Barness E, Kapur RP, Oligny LL, Siebert JR, editors. Potter's pathology of the fetus, infant and child. 2nd ed. Philadelphia: Mosby; 2007.
10. Cohen M, Scheimberg I, editors. The pediatric and perinatal autopsy manual. Cambridge: Cambridge University Press; 2000. https://doi.org/10.1017/CBO9781139237017.
11. Gripp K, Slavotinek A, Hall J, Allanson J. Handbook of physical measurements. Oxford: Oxford University Press; 2013.

12. Archie JG, Collins JS, Lebel RR. Quantitative standards for fetal and neonatal autopsy. Am J Clin Pathol. 2006;126(2):256–65.
13. Merlob P, Sivan Y, Reisner SH. Anthropometric measurements of the newborn infant (27 to 41 gestational weeks). Birth Defects Orig Artic Ser. 1984;20(7):1–52.
14. Omotade O. Facial measurements in the newborn (towards syndrome delineation). J Med Genet. 1990;27:358–62. https://doi.org/10.1136/jmg.27.6.358.
15. Perinatal Institute @ www.gestation.net.
16. Publications, charts and training recourses of Intergrowth-21 @https://intergrowth21.tghn.org/.

Pathological Assessment of Fetal Growth

Beata Hargitai

Standard Postmortem Tables and Charts of Normal Weights and Measurements

When analyzing an individual case, collected data have to be compared to the "normal value" for a particular gestational age. It is a long and almost philosophical debate what can be appreciated as normal—or does it exist at all in setting of postmortem material. Recently published data derived from social termination cases—12–20 weeks of gestation—is probably the nearest to the definition of normal and this model is suitable to minimize postmortem artifacts; however, it does not solve the dilemma for later gestation [1] (Tables 1 and 2).

B. Hargitai (✉)
West Midlands Perinatal Pathology, Birmingham Women's and Children's Hospital, Birmingham, UK
e-mail: Beata.Hargitai@nhs.net

© Springer Nature Switzerland AG 2021
J. Martinovic (ed.), *Practical Manual of Fetal Pathology*,
https://doi.org/10.1007/978-3-030-42492-3_5

Table 1 External, radiological, cerebellar dimensions of fetuses without detectable pathology from uncomplicated pregnancies following termination of pregnancy at 12th–20th weeks of gestation (Mean, standard deviation, number of cases)

GA (weeks)	External parameters (cm)							Radiological parameters (cm)					Brain dimension (mm)
	CRL	CFL	HC	TC	AC	Foot	Hand	BPD	FOD	T5	Humerus	Femur	Cerebellum
n	215	223	190	182	171	215	207	80	84	174	220	216	64
12	6.82 ± 0.73	8.85 ± 1.00	7.03 ± 0.69	5.97 ± 0.68	5.32 ± 0.76	0.90 ± 0.12	0.84 ± 0.14	2	2.72 ± 0.32	1.59 ± 0.15	0.71 ± 0.11	0.71 ± 0.12	9.9 ± 1.41
n	14	14	10	8	8	11	11	1	2	6	10	8	2
13	7.99 ± 0.78	11.11 ± 1.02	7.99 ± 0.82	6.72 ± 0.57	5.51 ± 0.72	1.15 ± 0.11	1.00 ± 0.11	2.24 ± 0.19	2.85 ± 0.23	1.85 ± 0.18	0.93 ± 0.13	0.89 ± 0.15	11.8 ± 0.49
n	43	44	36	33	32	44	42	14	16	36	46	45	7
14	9.51 ± 0.82	13.20 ± 1.19	9.20 ± 0.89	7.81 ± 0.62	6.56 ± 0.80	1.42 ± 0.19	1.27 ± 0.16	2.55 ± 0.19	3.31 ± 0.17	2.19 ± 0.16	1.25 ± 0.14	1.21 ± 0.15	13.01 ± 1.09
n	58	61	52	51	48	58	56	20	22	49	61	60	17
15	10.67 ± 0.83	15.34 ± 1.20	10.78 ± 1.21	9.08 ± 0.79	7.83 ± 1.36	1.72 ± 0.19	1.52 ± 0.19	3.04 ± 0.25	3.71 ± 0.24	2.47 ± 0.18	1.56 ± 0.15	1.55 ± 0.15	13.84 ± 0.88
n	35	37	32	32	28	35	35	15	17	30	37	37	10
16	11.53 ± 1.03	16.77 ± 1.21	12.01 ± 0.72	10.29 ± 0.66	8.42 ± 0.99	2.03 ± 0.12	1.75 ± 0.21	3.42 ± 0.20	4.19 ± 0.22	2.75 ± 0.15	1.85 ± 0.14	1.83 ± 0.15	14.96 ± 0.86
n	24	26	22	22	20	25	23	8	7	20	25	25	11
17	12.73 ± 0.55	18.55 ± 0.90	13.27 ± 0.79	11.11 ± 0.79	8.56 ± 1.05	2.34 ± 0.14	1.97 ± 0.16	3.63 ± 0.23	4.33 ± 0.28	2.98 ± 0.23	2.12 ± 0.13	2.13 ± 0.13	16.25 ± 0.88
n	20	20	18	16	16	21	19	13	6	13	20	20	8
18	13.89 ± 0.66	20.49 ± 0.65	14.58 ± 0.97	11.90 ± 0.88	9.45 ± 0.76	2.62 ± 0.21	2.32 ± 0.20	3.89 ± 0.22	4.93 ± 0.22	3.24 ± 0.25	2.41 ± 0.12	2.45 ± 0.17	17.65 ± 0.5
n	11	11	11	11	11	11	11	5	8	11	11	11	6
19	15.18 ± 0.71	22.88 ± 1.58	15.82 ± 1.35	12.64 ± 1.30	10.34 ± 1.30	2.95 ± 0.18	2.42 ± 0.08	4.30 ± 0.28	5.44 ± 0.32	3.40 ± 0.20	2.75 ± 0.12	2.90 ± 0.21	19.25 ± 0.35
n	6	6	5	5	5	6	6	2	4	6	6	6	2
20	16.67 ± 0.46	25.48 ± 1.23	16.88 ± 0.68	14.23 ± 0.13	11.97 ± 1.12	3.31 ± 0.18	2.72 ± 0.15	4.38 ± 0.04	5.93 ± 0.04	3.63 ± 0.08	3.00 ± 0.11	3.10 ± 0.14	20
n	4	6	4	4	3	4	4	2	2	3	4	4	1

AC abdominal circumference, *BPD* biparietal diameter, *cerebellum* transversal cerebellum diameter, *CFL* crown foot length, *CRL* crown rump length, *FOD* fronto-occipital diameter, *GA* gestational age, *HC* head circumference, *TC* thoracic circumference, *T5* thoracic diameter at the level of the fifth rib

Regression of data incorporating multiple sources produced valuable quantitative standards for the perinatal age group for linear body and facial measurements, body and organ weights—providing good alternative if local reference data are not available [2] (Tables 3 and 4). Further references on facial measurement standards have been published comparing results of several studies from various geographic regions [3, 4]. Foot length correlates well with age and if foot length is not available, hand length can be helpful—further tables and charts are included for reference (Table 5) (Figs. 1 and 2). Long bone measurement tables have been published based on ultrasound biometry [5] (Tables 6, 7, and 8).

Growth charts are preferably customized for gender, parity, maternal BMI, and ethnicity although there are arguments against significance of inclusion of maternal characteristics [6]. It has been recognized that in the present era and probably for the future, use of mixed-population based—instead of using ethnicity based—charts is the preferable choice, viewing the large and increasing proportion of mixed race, multi-ethnic population, especially in large cities of the world [7–9] (Fig. 3). Reference ranges for organ weights of infants were published by a large single center study [10] and standard tables are available for live born, preterm and term infants who subsequently died and were referred for postmortem investigation with diagnosis of sudden unexpected death of infancy [11].

For fetuses with appropriate growth for gestation (AGA), tables and charts showing organ weight against gestational age can be suitable. When there is evidence of impaired fetal growth, and ambiguity of the length of gestation, use of charts and tables showing organ weights against birth weight seems to be a better option. If growth restriction is suspected in a macerated baby, tables showing body weight and organ weights against the femur length are particularly useful, especially when gestational age could not be determined with full accuracy. Although it would be reasonable to use separate growth standards and organ weights for non-macerated and macerated cases, there is only a limited number of references (12). Customized tables of autopsy standards were designed at the West Midlands Perinatal Pathology, Birmingham UK, to help with these practical challenges (Tables 9, 10, 11, 12) (Figs. 4 and 5).

For cases of multiple gestation, use of customized twin charts is recommended [13] (Figs. 6 and 7).

As it was discussed in section "Obstetric Ultrasonographic Fetal Biometry," tables for body weight and body measurements can be obtained clinically, using ultrasound biometry of surviving babies, and similarly, organ weights can be estimated based on ultrasound scan.

Biometrical data, including organ weights, can be derived from traditional autopsy examination or using postmortem MRI [14, 15].

Table 2 Fetal and organ weights (g) of fetuses without detectable pathology from uncomplicated pregnancies following termination of pregnancy at 12th–20th weeks of gestation (Mean, standard deviation and number of cases)

GA (weeks)	Fetus	Brain	Heart	Lungs	Right lung	Left lung
n	203	145	160	177	115	115
12	17.86 ± 4.80	3.6 ± 2.03	0.15 ± 0.09	0.49 ± 0.24	–	–
n	12	5	6	7	–	–
13	28.11 ± 6.41	5.26 ± 1.14	0.21 ± 0.06	0.89 ± 0.29	0.45 ± 0.16	0.39 ± 0.14
n	41	25	29	33	17	17
14	45.88 ± 10.58	7.96 ± 2.03	0.33 ± 0.12	1.52 ± 0.43	0.81 ± 0.23	0.67 ± 0.2
n	57	43	41	49	31	31
15	69.41 ± 13.07	11.33 ± 2.21	0.46 ± 0.15	2.34 ± 0.58	1.23 ± 0.39	0.99 ± 0.3
n	32	21	29	29	17	17
16	98.60 ± 11.60	15.48 ± 3.19	0.64 ± 0.12	3.04 ± 0.55	1.69 ± 0.32	1.44 ± 0.25
n	25	19	18	20	17	17
17	125.21 ± 17.84	20.13 ± 2.62	0.80 ± 0.19	3.93 ± 0.61	2.13 ± 0.36	1.77 ± 0.29
n	15	15	18	19	16	16
18	172.04 ± 25.16	26.26 ± 4.48	1.14 ± 0.36	4.89 ± 0.76	2.67 ± 0.45	2.24 ± 0.35
n	11	11	11	11	10	10
19	228.47 ± 43.37	34.58 ± 5.02	1.65 ± 0.43	6.09 ± 0.25	3.37 ± 0.09	2.79 ± 0.14
n	6	4	5	6	5	5
20	306.50 ± 26.71	46.0 ± 0.57	1.99 ± 0.18	6.64 ± 1.15	3.63 ± 0.95	2.97 ± 0.74
n	4	2	3	3	2	2

GA gestational age

Thymus	Liver	Spleen	Kidneys	Right kidney	Left kidney	Adrenals	Placenta
106	151	111	163	93	93	151	196
0.07 ± 0.05	1.15 ± 0.43	0.05 ± 0.07	0.2 ± 0.13	–	–	0.10 ± 0.06	39.02 ± 42.32
3	5	2	5	–	–	5	9
0.03 ± 0.01	1.49 ± 0.30	0.03 ± 0.03	0.21 ± 0.07	0.1 ± 0.03	0.1 ± 0.03	0.14 ± 0.06	43.86 ± 14.91
11	25	13	29	9	9	22	35
0.08 ± 0.11	2.36 ± 0.52	0.05 ± 0.04	0.36 ± 0.13	0.18 ± 0.08	0.18 ± 0.07	0.25 ± 0.08	51.64 ± 21.53
23	45	26	42	25	25	41	54
0.09 ± 0.06	3.37 ± 0.66	0.07 ± 0.06	0.53 ± 0.15	0.25 ± 0.05	0.25 ± 0.06	0.35 ± 0.12	63.44 ± 17.18
21	25	21	28	12	12	27	33
0.12 ± 0.04	4.63 ± 0.78	0.09 ± 0.06	0.71 ± 0.19	0.35 ± 0.08	0.37 ± 0.1	0.44 ± 0.09	74.24 ± 18.09
15	19	17	19	16	16	19	25
0.22 ± 0.13	6.07 ± 1.07	0.10 ± 0.04	1.11 ± 0.33	0.55 ± 0.17	0.56 ± 0.17	0.61 ± 0.17	80.97 ± 24.08
16	14	14	19	14	14	18	20
0.24 ± 0.06	7.92 ± 1.21	0.15 ± 0.04	1.43 ± 0.20	0.7 ± 0.1	0.71 ± 0.11	0.90 ± 0.23	91.64 ± 16.91
10	10	9	11	10	10	10	11
0.35 ± 0.04	10.77 ± 1.45	0.20 ± 0.08	1.76 ± 0.51	0.88 ± 0.35	0.86 ± 0.29	1.05 ± 0.24	120.83 ± 29.96
4	5	6	6	4	4	6	6
0.45 ± 0.14	12.76 ± 1.23	0.35 ± 0.05	2.63 ± 0.63	1.22 ± 0.17	1.12 ± 0.16	1.27 ± 0.32	116.00 ± 22.98
3	3	3	4	3	3	3	4

Table 3 Expected linear measurements and SDs at various postmenstrual gestational ages[a]

Age (weeks)	CHL	CRL	HC	BPD	OCD	ICD	PL	CC	IND	AC	HL	FL	SIL	LIL
12	93.0 ± 9.7	76.1 ± 6.7	67.7 ± 11.6	19.5 ± 3.5	14.0 ± 4.0	6.04 ± 1.55	–	–	14.1 ± 3.4	–	–	9.74 ± 1.11	194	20
13	114 ± 11	86.7 ± 7.8	82.1 ± 11.7	23.2 ± 3.6	16.7 ± 4.0	6.93 ± 1.56	2.80	76.7	16.3 ± 3.5	59.8	11.3	12.3 ± 1.1	282	39
14	134 ± 12	97.7 ± 8.8	96.2 ± 11.9	26.8 ± 3.6	19.3 ± 4.0	7.80 ± 1.57	3.09	86.1	18.5 ± 3.7	68.9	13.7	15.1 ± 1.1	370	58
15	154 ± 14	109 ± 10	110 ± 12	30.4 ± 3.7	21.9 ± 4.0	8.64 ± 1.58	3.39	95.4	20.7 ± 3.9	78.0	16.1	17.9 ± 1.1	458	77
16	174 ± 15	121 ± 11	123 ± 12	33.9 ± 3.8	24.4 ± 4.0	9.45 ± 1.59	3.68	105	22.9 ± 4.1	87.2	18.6	20.9 ± 1.2	547	96
17	193 ± 16	133 ± 11	136 ± 12	37.3 ± 3.8	26.8 ± 4.0	10.2 ± 1.6	3.98	114	25.0 ± 4.3	96.3	21.0	24.0 ± 1.2	635	115
18	212 ± 17	145 ± 12	149 ± 13	40.7 ± 3.9	29.2 ± 4.0	11.0 ± 1.6	4.27	124	27.2 ± 4.4	105	23.4	27.2 ± 1.4	723	134
19	230 ± 18	158 ± 13	161 ± 13	43.9 ± 4.0	31.5 ± 4.1	11.7 ± 1.6	4.57	133	29.4 ± 4.6	115	25.8	30.5 ± 1.5	811	152
20	247 ± 19	171 ± 14	173 ± 13	47.1 ± 4.1	33.8 ± 4.1	12.5 ± 1.6	4.86	142	31.6 ± 4.8	124	28.2	33.9 ± 1.7	900	171
21	264 ± 19	184 ± 14	185 ± 13	50.2 ± 4.1	35.9 ± 4.1	13.1 ± 1.7	5.16	152	33.8 ± 5.0	133	30.6	37.2 ± 1.9	988	190
22	278 ± 20	195 ± 15	196 ± 13	53.3 ± 4.2	38.1 ± 4.1	13.8 ± 1.7	5.45	161	36.0 ± 5.1	142	32.9	40.0 ± 2.1	1076	209
23	291 ± 20	204 ± 15	207 ± 14	56.2 ± 4.3	40.1 ± 4.1	14.4 ± 1.7	5.75	170	38.2 ± 5.3	151	35.3	41.7 ± 2.4	1164	228
24	303 ± 21	213 ± 16	218 ± 14	59.1 ± 4.3	42.1 ± 4.1	15.0 ± 1.7	6.04	180	40.4 ± 5.5	160	37.8	43.8 ± 2.6	1253	247
25	316 ± 22	223 ± 17	228 ± 14	61.9 ± 4.4	44.0 ± 4.1	15.6 ± 1.7	6.33	189	42.6 ± 5.7	169	40.4	46.0 ± 3.0	1341	266
26	328 ± 23	232 ± 18	238 ± 14	64.7 ± 4.5	45.9 ± 4.1	16.2 ± 1.7	6.63	199	44.8 ± 5.8	179	43.0	48.0 ± 3.5	–	–
27	340 ± 26	242 ± 19	248 ± 14	67.3 ± 4.5	47.7 ± 4.2	16.7 ± 1.7	–	208	47.0 ± 6.0	–	45.7	50.0 ± 3.9	–	–
28	351 ± 30	250 ± 21	257 ± 14	69.9 ± 4.6	49.4 ± 4.2	17.2 ± 1.7	–	217	49.2 ± 6.2	–	48.4	52.0 ± 4.3	–	–
29	362 ± 33	259 ± 24	266 ± 15	72.4 ± 4.7	51.1 ± 4.2	17.7 ± 1.7	–	227	51.4 ± 6.4	–	51.0	54.1 ± 4.9	–	–
30	374 ± 35	267 ± 27	275 ± 15	74.8 ± 4.8	52.7 ± 4.2	18.1 ± 1.8	–	236	53.5 ± 6.6	–	53.4	56.2 ± 5.4	–	–
31	386 ± 37	276 ± 30	283 ± 15	77.2 ± 4.8	54.2 ± 4.2	18.6 ± 1.8	–	245	55.7 ± 6.7	–	55.6	58.2 ± 6.0	–	–
32	397 ± 38	284 ± 32	291 ± 15	79.4 ± 4.9	55.7 ± 4.2	19.0 ± 1.8	–	255	57.9 ± 6.9	–	576 ± 2.1	60.4 ± 6.3	–	–

Age (weeks)	CHL	CRL	HC	BPD	OCD	ICD	PL	CC	IND	AC	HL	FL	SIL	LIL
33	408 ± 40	292 ± 33	298 ± 15	81.6 ± 5.0	57.1 ± 4.2	19.3 ± 1.8	–	264	60.1 ± 7.1	–	59.2 ± 2.9	62.5 ± 6.4	–	–
34	419 ± 41	301 ± 33	306 ± 16	83.7 ± 5.0	58.5 ± 4.2	19.7 ± 1.8	–	274	62.3 ± 7.3	–	60.5 ± 4.1	64.7 ± 6.6	–	–
35	432 ± 43	310 ± 33	312 ± 16	85.8 ± 5.1	59.8 ± 4.2	20.0 ± 1.8	–	283	64.5 ± 7.4	–	61.9 ± 4.8	66.9 ± 6.7	–	–
36	444 ± 44	318 ± 33	319 ± 16	87.8 ± 5.2	61.0 ± 4.3	20.3 ± 1.8	–	292	66.7 ± 7.6	–	63.2 ± 5.1	69.2 ± 6.7	–	–
37	457 ± 44	327 ± 32	325 ± 16	89.6 ± 5.2	62.2 ± 4.3	20.6 ± 1.8	–	302	68.9 ± 7.8	–	64.4 ± 5.4	71.3 ± 6.7	–	–
38	470 ± 44	336 ± 32	331 ± 16	91.5 ± 5.3	63.3 ± 4.3	20.8 ± 1.9	–	311	71.1 ± 8.0	–	65.4 ± 5.5	73.4 ± 6.7	–	–
39	482 ± 44	344 ± 30	336 ± 17	93.2 ± 5.4	64.3 ± 4.3	21.0 ± 1.9	–	321	73.3 ± 8.1	–	66.3 ± 5.5	75.6 ± 6.7	–	–
40	493 ± 42	352 ± 29	342 ± 17	94.9 ± 5.5	65.3 ± 4.3	21.2 ± 1.9	–	330	75.5 ± 8.3	–	670 ± 5.3	77.8 ± 6.6	–	–
41	505 ± 41	360 ± 27	346 ± 17	96.4 ± 5.5	66.2 ± 4.3	21.4 ± 1.9	–	–	77.7 ± 8.5	–	676 ± 4.9	80.1 ± 6.4	–	–
42	516 ± 38	367 ± 25	351 ± 17	97.9 ± 5.6	67.0 ± 4.3	21.5 ± 1.9	–	–	79.9 ± 8.7	–	68.0 ± 4.2	82.5 ± 6.3	–	–

AC abdominal circumference, BPD biparietal diameter, CC chest circumference, CHL crown–heel length, CRL crown–rump length, FL foot length, HC head circumference, HL hand length, ICD inner canthal distance, IND internipple distance, LIL large intestine length, OCD outer canthal distance, PL philtrum length, SIL small intestine length

[a]Data are given as mean or mean ± SD. Linear measurements are given in millimeters

Table 4 Expected weights and SDs at various postmenstrual gestational ages[a]

Age (weeks)	Body	Brain	Thymus	Lungs	Heart	Liver	Spleen	Adrenals	Pancreas	Kidneys
12	20.9 ± 6.6	3.20 ± 1.44	0.01 ± 0.01	0.50 ± 0.28	0.15 ± 0.02	1.01 ± 0.38	0.01 ± 0.01	0.10 ± 0.03	–	0.16 ± 0.04
13	31.2 ± 10.1	5.19 ± 1.95	0.03 ± 0.01	1.08 ± 0.45	0.20 ± 0.06	1.38 ± 0.57	0.01 ± 0.01	0.15 ± 0.05	–	0.22 ± 0.07
14	49.1 ± 14.5	8.14 ± 2.58	0.05 ± 0.02	1.79 ± 0.67	0.31 ± 0.11	2.18 ± 0.84	0.03 ± 0.02	0.23 ± 0.08	–	0.36 ± 0.13
15	74.7 ± 19.8	12.0 ± 3.3	0.09 ± 0.04	2.64 ± 0.92	0.50 ± 0.17	3.41 ± 1.18	0.05 ± 0.03	0.33 ± 0.12	–	0.59 ± 0.19
16	108 ± 26	16.9 ± 4.2	0.14 ± 0.06	3.61 ± 1.21	0.76 ± 0.24	5.06 ± 1.60	0.09 ± 0.05	0.47 ± 0.16	–	0.90 ± 0.28
17	149 ± 33	22.8 ± 5.2	0.20 ± 0.08	4.70 ± 1.55	1.10 ± 0.31	7.14 ± 2.10	0.15 ± 0.07	0.64 ± 0.22	–	1.30 ± 0.39
18	197 ± 42	29.7 ± 6.3	0.28 ± 0.12	5.92 ± 1.92	1.50 ± 0.40	9.65 ± 2.66	0.21 ± 0.10	0.84 ± 0.30	–	1.79 ± 0.51
19	255 ± 51	37.2 ± 7.6	0.41 ± 0.17	7.30 ± 2.34	1.88 ± 0.49	12.8 ± 3.3	0.30 ± 0.14	1.03 ± 0.34	–	2.36 ± 0.65
20	319 ± 61	45.7 ± 8.9	0.54 ± 0.23	8.84 ± 2.80	2.41 ± 0.59	16.5 ± 4.0	0.41 ± 0.18	1.29 ± 0.41	0.50 ± 0.14	3.00 ± 0.81
21	389 ± 72	54.6 ± 10.4	0.72 ± 0.29	10.4 ± 3.3	2.89 ± 0.71	19.9 ± 4.8	0.54 ± 0.22	1.51 ± 0.49	0.54 ± 0.21	3.63 ± 0.99
22	452 ± 84	63.7 ± 12.0	0.92 ± 0.37	12.0 ± 3.8	3.38 ± 0.82	22.7 ± 5.7	0.66 ± 0.28	1.73 ± 0.57	0.60 ± 0.26	4.23 ± 1.18
23	510 ± 97	72.3 ± 13.8	1.15 ± 0.46	13.5 ± 4.4	3.81 ± 0.96	24.3 ± 6.5	0.75 ± 0.32	1.88 ± 0.66	0.68 ± 0.31	4.77 ± 1.39
24	579 ± 115	82.8 ± 15.6	1.38 ± 0.58	15.0 ± 5.0	4.23 ± 1.12	26.4 ± 7.1	0.91 ± 0.36	2.00 ± 0.74	0.77 ± 0.34	5.65 ± 1.63
25	660 ± 134	93.4 ± 17.4	1.63 ± 0.71	16.8 ± 5.6	4.80 ± 1.31	29.4 ± 7.8	1.11 ± 0.44	2.16 ± 0.82	0.85 ± 0.36	6.55 ± 1.91
26	744 ± 163	105 ± 19	1.96 ± 0.86	18.7 ± 6.2	5.50 ± 1.57	33.2 ± 8.8	1.38 ± 0.55	2.36 ± 0.90	0.92 ± 0.38	7.46 ± 2.21
27	839 ± 199	118 ± 21	2.37 ± 1.02	20.6 ± 6.8	6.28 ± 1.84	37.8 ± 9.9	1.78 ± 0.71	2.58 ± 0.99	1.01 ± 0.38	8.53 ± 2.53
28	946 ± 239	135 ± 24	2.85 ± 1.22	22.7 ± 7.3	7.13 ± 2.11	42.6 ± 11.5	2.26 ± 0.96	2.83 ± 1.10	1.08 ± 0.37	9.75 ± 2.85
29	1064 ± 286	154 ± 26	3.44 ± 1.49	25.1 ± 7.9	7.95 ± 2.44	46.9 ± 13.3	2.73 ± 1.19	3.09 ± 1.21	1.14 ± 0.37	11.1 ± 3.2
30	1211 ± 330	173 ± 30	4.02 ± 1.85	27.4 ± 8.4	8.84 ± 2.71	51.3 ± 14.8	3.20 ± 1.36	3.36 ± 1.34	1.27 ± 0.39	12.5 ± 3.7
31	1351 ± 373	191 ± 33	4.52 ± 2.17	29.2 ± 8.8	9.83 ± 2.86	55.9 ± 15.8	3.74 ± 1.58	3.71 ± 1.42	1.46 ± 0.42	13.8 ± 4.0

Age (weeks)	Body	Brain	Thymus	Lungs	Heart	Liver	Spleen	Adrenals	Pancreas	Kidneys
32	1492 ± 406	206 ± 35	4.91 ± 2.43	31.2 ± 9.0	10.8 ± 3.0	61.2 ± 17.0	4.37 ± 1.87	4.07 ± 1.50	1.77 ± 0.47	15.0 ± 4.4
33	1650 ± 433	222 ± 36	5.40 ± 2.63	34.1 ± 9.4	11.9 ± 3.2	66.3 ± 18.8	5.06 ± 2.18	4.42 ± 1.56	1.95 ± 0.55	16.5 ± 4.9
34	1832 ± 457	242 ± 37	6.03 ± 2.84	37.5 ± 10.1	13.1 ± 3.5	72.8 ± 20.9	5.76 ± 2.51	4.77 ± 1.63	2.11 ± 0.63	18.0 ± 5.3
35	2040 ± 487	265 ± 39	6.87 ± 3.06	41.7 ± 11.0	14.5 ± 3.7	81.8 ± 22.3	6.47 ± 2.79	5.19 ± 1.76	2.36 ± 0.69	19.6 ± 5.7
36	2246 ± 511	292 ± 42	7.85 ± 3.22	45.1 ± 12.2	16.0 ± 4.0	92.8 ± 22.9	7.21 ± 3.07	5.74 ± 1.92	2.61 ± 0.77	21.3 ± 6.0
37	2424 ± 535	319 ± 44	8.95 ± 3.41	47.0 ± 13.2	17.6 ± 4.3	104 ± 23	8.11 ± 3.30	6.46 ± 2.10	2.84 ± 0.85	22.5 ± 6.4
38	2603 ± 559	340 ± 46	9.61 ± 3.60	48.4 ± 14.0	18.6 ± 4.5	116 ± 26	9.15 ± 3.53	7.01 ± 2.31	3.04 ± 0.94	23.9 ± 6.8
39	2787 ± 582	355 ± 49	9.98 ± 3.78	49.4 ± 14.8	19.4 ± 4.8	124 ± 29	9.83 ± 3.73	7.44 ± 2.55	3.33 ± 1.04	24.9 ± 7.1
40	2942 ± 603	368 ± 51	10.2 ± 3.9	50.8 ± 15.5	20.3 ± 5.0	130 ± 32	10.2 ± 3.9	7.75 ± 2.82	3.65 ± 1.15	25.7 ± 7.5
41	3098 ± 623	382 ± 53	10.2 ± 4.1	52.3 ± 16.1	21.3 ± 5.2	136 ± 36	10.5 ± 4.0	7.99 ± 3.11	4.01 ± 1.26	26.4 ± 7.8
42	3267 ± 641	395 ± 55	10.1 ± 4.3	54.0 ± 16.5	22.4 ± 5.3	141 ± 40	10.8 ± 4.0	8.14 ± 3.44	4.40 ± 1.39	27.0 ± 8.2
43	3444 ± 657	408 ± 57	9.83 ± 4.46	55.9 ± 16.8	23.6 ± 5.4	145 ± 45	10.9 ± 4.0	8.21 ± 3.79	–	27.6 ± 8.5
44	3633 ± 671	421 ± 59	9.44 ± 4.64	57.8 ± 16.9	24.8 ± 5.5	149 ± 50	11.1 ± 4.0	8.22 ± 4.17	–	28.3 ± 8.8

[a]Lungs, adrenals, and kidneys were weighed in pairs. Data are given as mean ± SD. Weights are given in grams

Table 5 Hand and foot length for 11–18 gestational weeks

Developmental age (weeks)	Hand length (mm)	Foot length (mm)
11	10	12
	±2	±2
12	15	17
	±2	±3
13	18	19
	±1	±1
14	19	22
	±1	±2
15	20	25
	±3	±3
16	26	28
	±2	±2
17	27	29
	±3	±4
18	29	33
	±2	±2

After McBride et al. 1984 and Kalousek et al. 1990, with permission
From Gilbert-Barness E, Kapur RP, Oligny LL, Siebert JR (eds). Potter's Pathology of the Fetus, Infant and Child (2nd edition). Philadelphia: Mosby, 2007 with permission

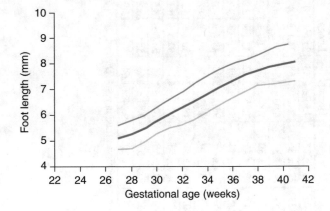

Fig. 1 Foot length for 27–42 weeks of gestation. (From Karen W Gripp et al: Handbook of Physical Measurements, printed by permission from Merlob 1984)

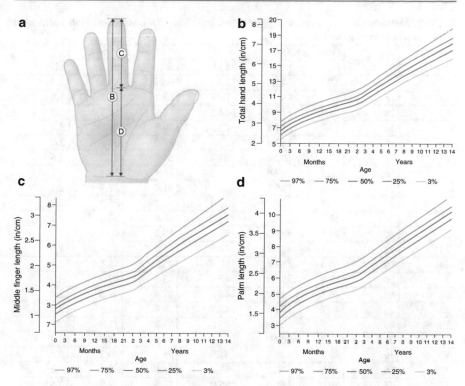

Fig. 2 Hand measurements. (From Karen W Gripp et al: Handbook of Physical Measurements, printed by permission from Merlob 1984)

Table 6 Measurements for humerus length (fitted 3rd, 10th, 50th, 90th, and 97th centiles) at 12–42 exact weeks of gestation

Weeks of gestation	n	Fitted centiles					SD
		3rd	10th	50th	90th	97th	
12	8	3.7	4.8	7.1	9.5	10.6	1.8
13	18	7.2	8.3	10.7	13.1	14.2	1.9
14	18	10.5	11.7	14.1	16.5	17.7	1.9
15	14	13.7	14.8	17.3	19.8	21.0	2.0
16	15	16.7	17.9	20.4	23.0	24.2	2.0
17	22	19.6	20.8	23.4	26.0	27.2	2.0
18	18	22.3	23.6	26.2	28.9	30.1	2.1
19	22	24.9	26.2	28.9	31.6	32.9	2.1
20	21	27.4	28.7	31.5	34.2	35.5	2.2
21	22	29.8	31.2	34.0	36.8	38.1	2.2
22	20	32.1	33.5	36.3	39.2	40.5	2.2
23	22	34.3	35.7	38.6	41.5	42.9	2.3
24	24	36.4	37.8	40.7	43.7	45.1	2.3
25	20	38.4	39.8	42.8	45.8	47.2	2.4
26	19	40.3	41.7	44.8	47.9	49.3	2.4
27	24	42.1	43.6	46.7	49.8	51.3	2.4
28	20	43.9	45.3	48.5	51.7	53.2	2.5
29	21	45.5	47.0	50.2	53.3	55.0	2.5
30	19	47.1	48.6	51.9	55.2	56.7	2.6
31	26	48.6	50.2	53.5	56.8	58.4	2.6
32	25	50.0	51.6	55.0	58.4	59.9	2.6
33	23	51.4	53.0	56.4	59.8	61.5	2.7
34	20	52.7	54.3	57.8	61.3	62.9	2.7
35	20	53.9	55.6	59.1	62.6	64.3	2.8
36	24	55.1	56.8	60.3	63.9	65.6	2.8
37	19	56.2	57.9	61.5	65.1	66.8	2.8
38	20	57.2	58.9	62.6	66.3	68.0	2.9
39	14	58.2	60.0	63.7	67.4	69 2	2.9
40	13	59.1	60.9	64.7	68.5	70.3	3.0
41	25	60.0	61.8	65.6	69.5	71.3	3.0
42	17	60.8	62.6	66.5	70.4	72.2	3.0
Total	613						

© RCOG 2002 *Br J Obstet Gynaecol* **109**, pp. 919–929

Table 7 Measurements for ulna length (fitted 3rd, 10th, 50th, 90th, and 97th centiles) at 12–42 exact weeks of gestation

Weeks of gestation	n	Fitted centiles					SD
		3rd	10th	50th	90th	97th	
12	6	3.9	5.0	7.3	9.6	10.7	1.8
13	13	6.2	7.3	9.6	12.0	13.1	1.8
14	15	8.8	9.9	12.4	14.8	15.9	1.9
15	12	11.6	12.8	15.3	17.8	18.9	1.9
16	11	14.5	15.7	18.2	20.8	22.0	2.0
17	18	17.3	18.6	21.2	23.8	25.0	2.0
18	16	20.1	21.4	24.0	26.7	28.0	2.1
19	24	22.8	24 0	26.8	29.5	30.8	2.1
20	22	25.3	26.6	29.4	32.2	33.5	2.2
21	20	27.8	29.1	32.0	34.8	36.2	2.2
22	20	30.1	31.4	34.4	37.3	38.7	2.3
23	21	32.3	33.7	36.6	39.6	41.0	2.3
24	21	34.3	35.8	38.8	41.9	43.3	2.4
25	22	36.3	37.8	40.9	44.0	45.5	2.4
26	20	38.2	39.7	42.8	46.0	47.5	2.5
27	24	39.9	41.5	44.7	47.9	49.5	2.5
28	20	41.6	43.2	46.5	49.8	51.3	2.6
29	21	43.2	44.8	48.2	51.5	53.1	2.6
30	20	44.7	46.3	49.8	53.2	54.8	2.7
31	27	46.2	47.8	51.3	54.8	56.4	2.7
32	25	47.5	49.2	52.7	56.3	58.0	2.8
33	23	48.8	50.5	54.1	57.7	59.4	2.8
34	17	50.0	51.8	55.4	59.1	60.8	2.9
35	21	51.2	53.0	56.7	60.4	62.2	2.9
36	20	52.3	54.1	57.9	61.7	63.5	3.0
37	19	53.4	55.2	59.1	62.9	64.7	3.0
38	17	54.4	56.2	60.2	64.1	65.9	3.1
39	12	55.4	57.2	61.2	65.2	67.1	3.1
40	11	56.3	58.2	62.2	66.3	68.2	3.2
41	20	57.2	59.1	63.2	67.3	69.3	3.2
42	14	58.0	60.0	64.1	68.3	70.3	3.3
Total	572						

Table 8 Measurements for femur length (fitted 3rd, 10th, 50th, 90th, and 97th centiles) at 12–42 exact weeks of gestation

Weeks of gestation	n	Fitted centiles					SD
		3rd	10th	50th	90th	97th	
12	10	4.4	5.5	7.7	10.0	11.1	1.8
13	18	7.5	8.6	10.9	13.3	14.4	1.8
14	18	10.6	11.7	14.1	16.5	17.6	1.9
15	15	13.6	14.7	17.2	19.7	20.8	1.9
16	20	16.5	17.7	20.3	22.8	24.0	2.0
17	23	19.4	20.7	23.3	25.9	27.2	2.1
18	20	22.3	23.6	26.3	29.0	30.2	2.1
19	25	25.1	26.4	29.2	32.0	33.3	2.2
20	22	27.9	29.2	32.1	34.9	36.3	2.2
21	23	30.6	32.0	34.9	37.8	39.2	2.3
22	22	33.2	34.6	37.6	40.6	42.0	2.3
23	22	35.8	37.2	40.3	43.4	44.8	2.4
24	25	38.3	39.8	42.9	46.1	47.6	2.5
25	22	40.8	42.3	45.5	48.7	50.2	2.5
26	22	43.1	44.7	48.0	51.3	52.8	2.6
27	24	45.4	47.0	50.4	53.8	55.3	2.6
28	20	47.6	49.3	52.7	56.2	57.8	2.7
29	22	49.8	51.4	55.0	58.5	60.1	2.8
30	21	51.8	53.5	57.1	60.7	62.4	2.8
31	27	53.8	55.5	59.2	62.9	64.6	2.9
32	26	55.7	57.4	61.2	64.9	66.7	2.9
33	23	57.5	59.3	63.1	66.9	68.7	3.0
34	20	59.2	61.0	64.9	68.8	70.6	3.0
35	22	60.8	62.6	66.6	70.6	72.4	3.1
36	25	62.3	64.2	68.2	72.3	74.1	3.2
37	19	63.7	65.6	69.7	73.8	75.8	3.2
38	21	64.9	66.9	71.1	75.3	77.3	3.3
39	14	66.1	68.1	72.4	76.7	78.7	3.3
40	15	67.2	69.2	73.6	77.9	79.9	3.4
41	26	68.1	70.2	74.6	79.0	81.1	3.5
42	17	69.0	71.1	75.6	80.1	82.2	3.5
Total	649						

© RCOG 2002 *Br J Obstet Gynaecol* **109**, pp. 919–929

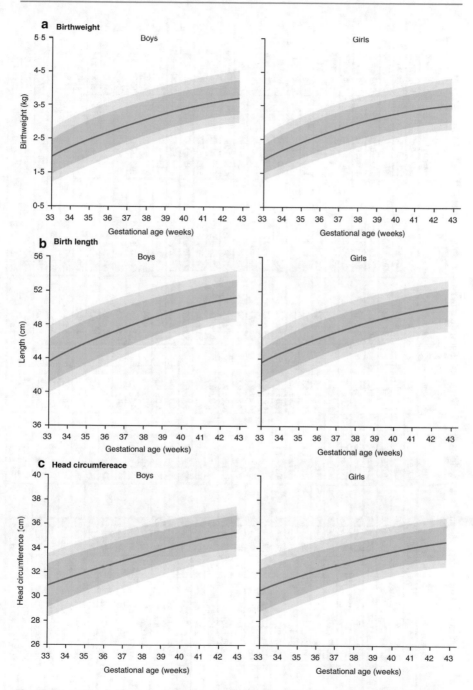

Fig. 3 International Newborn Size Standards. (Lancet. 2014 Sep 6;384(9946):857–68. doi: 10.1016/S0140-6736(14)60932-6. International standards for newborn weight, length, and head circumference by gestational age and sex: the Newborn Cross-Sectional Study of the INTERGROWTH-21st Project. Villar et al with permission)

Table 9 Postmortem external measurements and organ weights for 12–42 weeks of gestation in non-macerated fetuses (BWCH data)

Weeks of gestation	Body weight (g)	CHL (cm)	CRL (cm)	Foot (cm)	Femur (cm)	Brain (g)	Heart (g)	Left lung (g)
12	13.96 ± 5.65	9.5 ± 1.3	7.2 ± 1.0	0.9 ± 0.2	0.7 ± 0.2	2.62 ± 0.79	0.12 ± 0.05	0.19 ± 0.09
13	22.48 ± 9.91	11.5 ± 1.6	8.5 ± 1.1	1.1 ± 0.2	1.1 ± 0.2	5.04 ± 2.46	0.2 ± 0.08	0.3 ± 0.15
14	38.74 ± 12.37	13.6 ± 1.6	10.0 ± 1.1	1.4 ± 0.2	1.3 ± 0.2	8.03 ± 3.3	0.28 ± 0.1	0.61 ± 0.26
15	59.45 ± 17.42	15.7 ± 1.2	11.4 ± 0.9	1.6 ± 0.2	1.6 ± 0.2	11.81 ± 3.6	0.42 ± 0.15	0.93 ± 0.39
16	87.79 ± 22.29	17.4 ± 1.4	12.5 ± 1.1	1.9 ± 0.3	1.9 ± 0.2	16.81 ± 4.18	0.57 ± 0.15	1.58 ± 1.15
17	125.77 ± 27.76	19.2 ± 1.4	13.6 ± 1.0	2.1 ± 0.3	2.2 ± 0.2	22.15 ± 5.03	0.84 ± 0.23	2.08 ± 0.64
18	176.92 ± 23.27	21.4 ± 1.3	14.9 ± 0.9	2.6 ± 0.2	2.6 ± 0.2	30.39 ± 4.34	1.21 ± 0.23	2.61 ± 0.86
19	210.35 ± 52.38	22.9 ± 1.5	16.0 ± 1.1	2.8 ± 0.4	2.8 ± 0.2	36.52 ± 7.17	1.45 ± 0.38	2.8 ± 1.16
20	290.02 ± 45.29	25.4 ± 1.5	17.6 ± 1.1	3.3 ± 0.2	3.2 ± 0.2	49.58 ± 9.5	1.96 ± 0.42	3.65 ± 1.06
21	356.9 ± 46.12	26.7 ± 1.3	18.5 ± 1.1	3.5 ± 0.3	3.5 ± 0.2	55.57 ± 6.75	2.37 ± 0.51	4.64 ± 1.47
22	429.07 ± 52.94	28.4 ± 1.2	20.0 ± 1.5	3.8 ± 0.4	3.7 ± 0.2	68.23 ± 7.77	2.95 ± 0.51	5.4 ± 1.68
23	475.13 ± 80.66	29.9 ± 1.9	20.7 ± 1.5	4.0 ± 0.3	3.9 ± 0.3	78.55 ± 11.72	3.05 ± 0.76	4.99 ± 1.76
24	526.83 ± 107.93	30.8 ± 1.9	21.7 ± 1.2	4.1 ± 0.4	4.0 ± 0.3	83.4 ± 14.78	3.32 ± 0.88	5.28 ± 2.12
25	680.75 ± 111.29	33.6 ± 1.4	23.7 ± 1.0	4.5 ± 0.3	4.4 ± 0.2	113.36 ± 15.02	4.2 ± 0.93	6.81 ± 2.03
26	688.92 ± 164.4	33.7 ± 2.0	23.8 ± 1.5	4.7 ± 0.4	4.5 ± 0.3	106.64 ± 23.03	4.2 ± 1.08	5.41 ± 1.56
27	784.88 ± 167.27	35.4 ± 2.8	25.0 ± 1.7	5.0 ± 0.4	4.7 ± 0.4	129.38 ± 22.09	4.37 ± 1.41	7.48 ± 2.52
28	965.11 ± 211.36	37.5 ± 3.2	26.7 ± 2.4	5.2 ± 0.5	5.1 ± 0.3	141.55 ± 22.2	5.78 ± 1.67	8.01 ± 1.94
29	1080.12 ± 217.36	38.6 ± 2.2	27.1 ± 1.9	5.5 ± 0.6	5.3 ± 0.3	172.79 ± 36.06	6.45 ± 1.47	9.62 ± 2.75
30	1382.32 ± 178.96	41.7 ± 2.2	29.5 ± 1.9	6.0 ± 0.3	5.7 ± 0.4	198.09 ± 21.51	8.54 ± 2.52	12.81 ± 4.07
31	1494.5 ± 185.18	41.7 ± 2.2	29.2 ± 1.5	6.2 ± 0.5	5.8 ± 0.3	218.58 ± 35.41	8.86 ± 1.4	15.43 ± 3.98
32	1637.07 ± 220.59	43.9 ± 2.0	30.5 ± 2.4	6.0 ± 0.6	6.1 ± 0.4	216.57 ± 23.92	9.79 ± 2.03	15.02 ± 4.57
33	1805.3 ± 338.65	44.8 ± 2.5	31.3 ± 1.5	6.5 ± 0.5	6.3 ± 0.3	247.97 ± 26.75	10.3 ± 2.25	16.72 ± 5.68
34	2031.84 ± 370.86	45.4 ± 2.4	32.6 ± 1.8	7.0 ± 0.4	6.5 ± 0.3	277.44 ± 27.01	12.1 ± 2.65	19.3 ± 3.72
35	2148.89 ± 381.61	46.4 ± 2.2	32.9 ± 1.9	6.8 ± 0.7	6.6 ± 0.3	294.87 ± 36.49	12.75 ± 2.68	19.03 ± 4.26
36	2357.39 ± 371.37	48.2 ± 2.4	34.0 ± 2.1	7.1 ± 0.5	6.9 ± 0.3	303.8 ± 47.97	13.64 ± 2.68	21.5 ± 5.11
37	2539.89 ± 445.71	48.2 ± 2.5	34.9 ± 2.2	7.4 ± 0.5	7.1 ± 0.4	336.25 ± 45.77	14.82 ± 3.02	22.22 ± 5.65
38	2954.15 ± 405.67	50.3 ± 2.5	36.2 ± 1.6	7.6 ± 0.6	7.3 ± 0.4	363.47 ± 47.91	17.55 ± 3.61	23.91 ± 4.51
39	3036.25 ± 369.09	50.5 ± 2.4	36.6 ± 1.6	7.6 ± 0.5	7.5 ± 0.3	382.18 ± 29.59	18.0 ± 2.68	26.09 ± 5.51
40	3270.92 ± 363.71	51.5 ± 2.2	37.4 ± 1.3	7.9 ± 0.4	7.8 ± 0.3	404.36 ± 31.58	18.76 ± 3.25	27.69 ± 6.16
41	3358.81 ± 460.04	51.8 ± 2.3	37.6 ± 1.7	8.1 ± 0.4	7.9 ± 0.3	411.47 ± 43.44	19.24 ± 4.22	27.11 ± 5.47
42	3483.14 ± 602.16	51.7 ± 2.2	37.6 ± 2.7	8.3 ± 0.4	7.9 ± 0.3	393.89 ± 37.51	19.04 ± 1.76	27.62 ± 5.0

Right lung (g)	Lung combined (g)	Left kidney (g)	Right kidney (g)	Kidney combined (g)	Liver (g)	Adrenal combined (g)	Spleen (g)	Thymus (g)
0.2 ± 0.09	0.41 ± 0.21	0.09 ± 0.05	0.07 ± 0.05	0.12 ± 0.06	0.86 ± 0.38	0.09 ± 0.05	Missing data[a]	Missing data[a]
0.35 ± 0.17	0.67 ± 0.34	0.09 ± 0.05	0.11 ± 0.08	0.18 ± 0.1	1.29 ± 0.53	0.15 ± 0.09	0.05 ± 0.05	0.04 ± 0.02
0.68 ± 0.29	1.29 ± 0.53	0.17 ± 0.08	0.16 ± 0.07	0.33 ± 0.15	2.07 ± 0.87	0.21 ± 0.09	0.04 ± 0.02	0.05 ± 0.03
1.15 ± 0.46	2.12 ± 0.85	0.22 ± 0.07	0.23 ± 0.09	0.46 ± 0.18	2.92 ± 1.25	0.31 ± 0.15	0.06 ± 0.03	0.08 ± 0.04
1.88 ± 1.45	3.39 ± 2.5	0.38 ± 0.17	0.37 ± 0.17	0.72 ± 0.3	4.69 ± 1.97	0.46 ± 0.21	0.09 ± 0.04	0.09 ± 0.04
2.45 ± 0.76	4.51 ± 1.42	0.56 ± 0.17	0.53 ± 0.14	1.08 ± 0.33	6.88 ± 3.05	0.62 ± 0.26	0.13 ± 0.06	0.15 ± 0.07
3.15 ± 1.0	5.91 ± 1.89	0.83 ± 0.25	0.79 ± 0.25	1.63 ± 0.44	9.98 ± 3.15	0.92 ± 0.35	0.18 ± 0.07	0.21 ± 0.08
3.43 ± 1.36	6.39 ± 2.45	1.03 ± 0.36	1.04 ± 0.36	2.01 ± 0.62	11.71 ± 4.37	1.04 ± 0.47	0.27 ± 0.12	0.28 ± 0.14
4.49 ± 1.25	8.08 ± 2.19	1.36 ± 0.26	1.4 ± 0.36	2.73 ± 0.56	16.59 ± 5.0	1.36 ± 0.55	0.37 ± 0.14	0.43 ± 0.21
5.7 ± 1.87	10.15 ± 3.09	1.65 ± 0.54	1.61 ± 0.49	3.24 ± 0.84	20.5 ± 5.12	1.6 ± 0.52	0.5 ± 0.18	0.66 ± 0.24
6.63 ± 2.13	12.02 ± 3.72	2.11 ± 0.59	2.04 ± 0.56	4.06 ± 1.12	23.79 ± 7.52	1.87 ± 0.68	0.66 ± 0.4	0.75 ± 0.37
6.15 ± 2.35	11.11 ± 4.04	2.09 ± 0.79	2.01 ± 0.71	4.04 ± 1.34	22.04 ± 8.85	1.75 ± 0.65	0.61 ± 0.25	0.69 ± 0.38
6.33 ± 2.59	11.61 ± 4.54	2.13 ± 0.89	2.25 ± 0.96	4.42 ± 1.76	24.81 ± 11.16	1.88 ± 0.75	0.76 ± 0.29	0.83 ± 0.38
8.52 ± 2.46	15.25 ± 4.39	3.45 ± 1.0	3.28 ± 0.95	5.97 ± 1.87	27.81 ± 12.27	2.07 ± 0.78	1.08 ± 0.41	1.18 ± 0.73
6.8 ± 1.92	13.32 ± 4.57	3.28 ± 1.37	3.18 ± 1.37	6.28 ± 2.41	30.19 ± 15.82	2.05 ± 0.76	1.11 ± 0.52	1.13 ± 0.67
9.95 ± 3.28	17.38 ± 5.22	3.38 ± 1.68	3.18 ± 1.33	6.37 ± 2.53	26.81 ± 11.09	1.86 ± 0.83	1.53 ± 0.67	1.48 ± 0.94
9.96 ± 2.81	17.89 ± 4.63	3.73 ± 1.37	4.07 ± 1.59	8.05 ± 2.44	34.62 ± 12.93	2.32 ± 0.95	1.68 ± 0.85	1.81 ± 0.83
12.13 ± 3.12	21.36 ± 5.66	5.2 ± 2.05	5.15 ± 1.8	9.41 ± 2.58	37.16 ± 12.19	2.75 ± 0.9	1.99 ± 0.87	1.88 ± 0.89
15.76 ± 5.07	28.85 ± 8.98	6.9 ± 1.42	7.17 ± 1.72	12.72 ± 3.59	58.12 ± 24.31	3.78 ± 1.02	3.31 ± 1.74	3.09 ± 1.46
19.76 ± 5.1	34.97 ± 8.78	6.6 ± 1.68	6.82 ± 2.05	13.86 ± 3.69	60.34 ± 17.75	3.88 ± 0.79	3.71 ± 1.49	3.66 ± 1.64
19.21 ± 5.51	33.55 ± 9.43	8.06 ± 2.03	8.07 ± 2.34	15.54 ± 4.42	62.32 ± 16.91	4.23 ± 1.42	4.83 ± 1.79	3.84 ± 2.29
20.89 ± 7.36	37.93 ± 12.68	7.83 ± 1.87	7.51 ± 1.37	15.38 ± 3.46	74.66 ± 24.44	4.69 ± 1.12	4.7 ± 1.44	5.39 ± 2.72
24.99 ± 4.91	44.48 ± 8.51	9.43 ± 2.72	9.49 ± 2.8	18.41 ± 5.65	85.91 ± 30.99	5.92 ± 2.82	4.91 ± 1.24	5.34 ± 2.51
24.67 ± 5.65	43.58 ± 10.78	10.3 ± 2.44	10.01 ± 2.69	19.74 ± 4.77	79.58 ± 25.65	4.94 ± 1.31	5.95 ± 2.24	6.28 ± 3.37
27.18 ± 6.36	47.55 ± 10.56	13.06 ± 4.66	12.52 ± 4.2	22.98 ± 6.55	89.53 ± 28.36	6.1 ± 2.17	6.65 ± 2.41	7.55 ± 4.39
26.77 ± 6.76	50.67 ± 12.76	10.55 ± 4.13	10.01 ± 3.56	20.57 ± 7.36	98.53 ± 35.38	6.82 ± 2.22	7.33 ± 3.16	7.64 ± 3.7
30.84 ± 7.25	55.21 ± 10.7	13.35 ± 3.65	13.31 ± 4.16	25.85 ± 7.25	115.98 ± 41.86	7.73 ± 2.66	8.33 ± 2.92	8.65 ± 4.15
32.6 ± 7.05	57.38 ± 12.7	13.56 ± 2.5	13.94 ± 2.44	26.08 ± 4.29	114.43 ± 33.78	7.75 ± 2.16	9.25 ± 3.25	8.6 ± 3.99
35.1 ± 8.06	63.37 ± 14.08	13.93 ± 3.55	13.46 ± 3.35	27.09 ± 6.51	138.38 ± 43.24	8.93 ± 2.13	11.56 ± 4.38	9.14 ± 2.93
33.95 ± 7.04	61.17 ± 12.2	15.35 ± 3.1	14.98 ± 2.72	28.18 ± 5.46	149.42 ± 50.05	9.32 ± 2.54	11.47 ± 3.19	9.51 ± 4.0
34.27 ± 5.16	60.19 ± 10.22	11.88 ± 1.86	12.33 ± 0.38	24.03 ± 6.25	159.94 ± 19.21	8.78 ± 3.06	13.79 ± 5.33	9.9 ± 1.69

[a]Insufficient number of valuables for analysis

Table 10 Postmortem external measurements and organ weights for 12–42 weeks of gestation in macerated fetuses (BWCH data)

Weeks of gestation	Body weight (g)	CHL (cm)	CRL (cm)	Foot (cm)	Femur (cm)	Brain (g)	Heart (g)	Left lung (g)
12	14.73 ± 7.1	9.9 ± 1.5	7.4 ± 1.0	0.9 ± 0.2	0.9 ± 0.2	2.76 ± 2.02	0.13 ± 0.06	0.17 ± 0.11
13	23.79 ± 9.07	11.9 ± 1.4	8.8 ± 1.1	1.1 ± 0.2	1.1 ± 0.2	5.07 ± 2.23	0.2 ± 0.09	0.35 ± 0.16
14	38.03 ± 12.15	14.1 ± 1.3	10.2 ± 1.1	1.4 ± 0.2	1.5 ± 0.2	7.29 ± 2.77	0.29 ± 0.1	0.55 ± 0.22
15	53.43 ± 15.66	15.8 ± 1.4	11.4 ± 1.0	1.5 ± 0.3	1.7 ± 0.2	11.77 ± 5.41	0.39 ± 0.12	0.82 ± 0.32
16	75.99 ± 25.43	17.6 ± 1.3	12.5 ± 1.0	1.8 ± 0.3	2.0 ± 0.2	15.48 ± 4.75	0.54 ± 0.18	1.09 ± 0.43
17	104.08 ± 31.6	19.4 ± 1.8	13.5 ± 1.9	2.0 ± 0.3	2.2 ± 0.3	21.89 ± 7.55	0.68 ± 0.23	1.33 ± 0.46
18	136.28 ± 40.64	21.0 ± 2.0	15.0 ± 1.2	2.3 ± 0.3	2.5 ± 0.3	28.54 ± 8.0	0.87 ± 0.29	1.6 ± 0.84
19	188.47 ± 54.26	23.3 ± 1.7	16.3 ± 1.3	2.7 ± 0.4	2.8 ± 0.2	40.87 ± 10.71	1.2 ± 0.38	2.21 ± 1.01
20	221.5 ± 76.21	23.9 ± 3.2	17.1 ± 1.8	3.0 ± 0.5	3.0 ± 0.4	38.58 ± 14.21	1.46 ± 0.51	2.39 ± 1.1
21	268.05 ± 78.59	27.1 ± 2.1	18.6 ± 1.8	3.3 ± 0.4	3.4 ± 0.3	53.43 ± 12.46	1.79 ± 0.52	2.32 ± 0.83
22	344.5 ± 65.4	28.2 ± 1.9	19.7 ± 1.5	3.6 ± 0.3	3.6 ± 0.3	61.88 ± 14.23	2.03 ± 0.58	2.79 ± 1.14
23	396.95 ± 72.2	29.8 ± 2.1	20.8 ± 1.6	3.7 ± 0.4	3.9 ± 0.3	68.68 ± 15.89	2.82 ± 0.73	3.69 ± 1.05
24	461.78 ± 118.09	30.7 ± 1.8	21.6 ± 1.4	4.0 ± 0.3	4.0 ± 0.3	81.58 ± 14.11	2.87 ± 0.82	3.78 ± 1.37
25	524.0 ± 177.58	31.2 ± 3.4	21.9 ± 2.4	4.1 ± 0.5	4.1 ± 0.6	81.38 ± 22.3	2.9 ± 1.04	3.88 ± 1.93
26	681.09 ± 181.55	34.7 ± 2.6	24.6 ± 2.2	4.6 ± 0.4	4.6 ± 0.4	114.11 ± 20.59	3.64 ± 1.08	5.29 ± 2.51
27	805.96 ± 155.49	36.1 ± 2.0	25.0 ± 2.0	5.0 ± 0.3	4.8 ± 0.3	125.87 ± 27.66	4.93 ± 1.4	7.01 ± 1.75
28	971.0 ± 164.35	37.7 ± 2.2	26.6 ± 1.4	5.2 ± 0.5	5.0 ± 0.3	138.1 ± 27.6	5.87 ± 1.57	8.39 ± 2.15
29	1104.32 ± 300.32	39.3 ± 3.3	27.5 ± 2.3	5.4 ± 0.5	5.2 ± 0.3	148.77 ± 31.32	6.18 ± 2.25	8.45 ± 3.63
30	1166.97 ± 215.4	39.4 ± 2.3	28.2 ± 1.8	5.6 ± 0.4	5.3 ± 0.4	174.71 ± 35.79	8.21 ± 2.12	11.17 ± 3.64
31	1331.67 ± 184.79	42.9 ± 2.6	30.0 ± 2.0	5.8 ± 0.4	5.7 ± 0.3	180.72 ± 22.52	7.96 ± 2.76	10.7 ± 4.05
32	1553.38 ± 307.81	42.3 ± 3.0	29.9 ± 2.1	5.8 ± 0.6	5.9 ± 0.4	196.16 ± 25.93	9.73 ± 4.54	12.86 ± 6.0
33	1768.38 ± 249.56	46.1 ± 1.8	32.5 ± 2.0	6.5 ± 0.4	6.3 ± 0.3	252.09 ± 29.83	9.81 ± 1.86	15.46 ± 4.56
34	2123.3 ± 421.93	46.1 ± 1.9	32.3 ± 2.4	6.7 ± 0.4	6.5 ± 0.3	258.46 ± 39.93	13.24 ± 2.34	17.57 ± 4.22
35	2310.48 ± 420.86	47.1 ± 2.0	33.8 ± 2.7	7.1 ± 0.5	6.7 ± 0.2	293.0 ± 48.57	12.29 ± 1.97	20.2 ± 7.73
36	2620.0 ± 586.5	48.8 ± 2.7	35.2 ± 2.1	7.2 ± 0.5	6.9 ± 0.3	311.9 ± 40.79	14.43 ± 2.95	20.13 ± 6.32
37	2644.29 ± 430.39	50.0 ± 2.5	35.7 ± 2.5	7.6 ± 0.4	7.2 ± 0.3	341.45 ± 32.12	15.39 ± 3.21	21.54 ± 5.3
38	2841.67 ± 441.63	49.8 ± 2.5	35.7 ± 2.0	7.3 ± 0.5	7.3 ± 0.4	343.19 ± 36.88	16.78 ± 4.54	23.31 ± 5.12
39	2995.65 ± 443.56	51.3 ± 2.5	36.8 ± 1.3	7.5 ± 0.5	7.5 ± 0.4	381.35 ± 37.25	16.33 ± 2.25	22.71 ± 4.73
40	3113.08 ± 471.82	51.2 ± 2.7	37.3 ± 2.1	7.7 ± 0.4	7.7 ± 0.3	393.97 ± 27.16	18.38 ± 4.97	26.1 ± 6.64
41	3298.25 ± 434.03	53.3 ± 2.3	38.5 ± 2.2	8.0 ± 0.4	7.9 ± 0.3	410.92 ± 50.61	18.87 ± 5.23	25.57 ± 4.08
42	2764.59 ± 1934.58	54.4 ± 3.3	40.8 ± 2.1	5.9 ± 3.5	6.1 ± 3.5	406.0 ± 90.18	21.75 ± 4.75	30.16 ± 3.33

Right lung (g)	Lung combined (g)	Left kidney (g)	Right kidney (g)	Kidney combined (g)	Liver (g)	Adrenal combined (g)	Spleen (g)	Thymus (g)
0.21 ± 0.13	0.47 ± 0.34	0.07 ± 0.04	0.06 ± 0.04	0.12 ± 0.06	0.93 ± 0.55	0.09 ± 0.05	0.04 ± 0.05	0.04 ± 0.03
0.44 ± 0.26	0.78 ± 0.41	0.08 ± 0.03	0.09 ± 0.04	0.16 ± 0.07	1.29 ± 0.57	0.13 ± 0.06	0.03 ± 0.01	0.04 ± 0.02
0.67 ± 0.26	1.18 ± 0.44	0.16 ± 0.07	0.16 ± 0.08	0.26 ± 0.11	1.86 ± 0.73	0.19 ± 0.08	0.05 ± 0.03	0.04 ± 0.03
0.98 ± 0.38	1.65 ± 0.69	0.2 ± 0.07	0.2 ± 0.08	0.37 ± 0.14	2.25 ± 0.84	0.28 ± 0.11	0.07 ± 0.03	0.06 ± 0.03
1.32 ± 0.48	2.34 ± 0.93	0.26 ± 0.1	0.28 ± 0.14	0.53 ± 0.22	2.84 ± 1.19	0.34 ± 0.13	0.08 ± 0.04	0.08 ± 0.04
1.53 ± 0.66	2.84 ± 1.18	0.36 ± 0.14	0.36 ± 0.16	0.67 ± 0.32	3.36 ± 1.72	0.41 ± 0.16	0.13 ± 0.15	0.1 ± 0.06
1.9 ± 1.03	3.47 ± 1.78	0.56 ± 0.18	0.55 ± 0.18	1.02 ± 0.46	4.61 ± 1.92	0.52 ± 0.23	0.15 ± 0.06	0.13 ± 0.06
2.65 ± 1.15	4.76 ± 1.97	0.82 ± 0.3	0.79 ± 0.32	1.43 ± 0.85	6.24 ± 2.82	0.67 ± 0.25	0.22 ± 0.12	0.19 ± 0.12
3.01 ± 1.36	5.34 ± 2.35	0.97 ± 0.3	0.97 ± 0.28	1.74 ± 0.75	8.8 ± 5.11	0.82 ± 0.42	0.28 ± 0.14	0.25 ± 0.14
2.95 ± 0.98	6.04 ± 2.02	0.91 ± 0.25	0.94 ± 0.16	1.94 ± 0.65	8.49 ± 3.74	0.96 ± 0.33	0.3 ± 0.15	0.27 ± 0.14
3.49 ± 1.4	6.33 ± 2.66	1.03 ± 0.31	1.18 ± 0.41	2.17 ± 0.74	11.18 ± 3.81	1.04 ± 0.41	0.4 ± 0.19	0.4 ± 0.25
4.56 ± 1.37	8.19 ± 2.38	1.44 ± 0.54	1.47 ± 0.49	3.08 ± 1.03	13.3 ± 5.73	1.16 ± 0.45	0.49 ± 0.26	0.46 ± 0.26
4.81 ± 1.74	8.82 ± 3.15	1.77 ± 0.54	1.77 ± 0.64	3.44 ± 1.35	14.95 ± 6.5	1.49 ± 0.67	0.66 ± 0.3	0.54 ± 0.27
4.67 ± 2.15	8.18 ± 3.46	1.93 ± 0.69	1.96 ± 0.69	4.19 ± 1.57	15.35 ± 7.09	1.26 ± 0.55	0.59 ± 0.35	0.54 ± 0.32
6.46 ± 2.8	12.26 ± 3.94	2.77 ± 0.98	2.64 ± 0.8	4.99 ± 1.7	17.97 ± 7.09	1.81 ± 0.69	1.16 ± 0.63	0.99 ± 0.43
8.91 ± 2.08	15.81 ± 3.66	3.21 ± 0.94	3.16 ± 0.76	6.21 ± 1.9	24.76 ± 7.69	1.95 ± 0.77	1.59 ± 0.65	1.22 ± 0.52
10.5 ± 2.51	18.41 ± 4.54	4.68 ± 0.9	4.98 ± 1.27	7.85 ± 2.4	34.38 ± 13.15	2.3 ± 0.52	1.82 ± 0.96	1.77 ± 0.95
10.75 ± 4.77	20.09 ± 7.37	5.32 ± 1.27	5.11 ± 1.27	8.78 ± 3.25	32.1 ± 14.37	2.44 ± 1.0	2.16 ± 1.3	1.67 ± 0.99
14.11 ± 4.33	24.6 ± 8.08	5.92 ± 1.55	6.29 ± 1.69	12.59 ± 3.56	44.83 ± 15.82	2.89 ± 0.91	2.45 ± 1.18	2.04 ± 1.22
12.67 ± 3.85	21.81 ± 6.78	4.65 ± 1.98	5.11 ± 2.03	9.43 ± 3.09	38.72 ± 14.25	2.76 ± 1.03	2.32 ± 0.91	1.89 ± 1.1
14.7 ± 4.59	26.43 ± 7.56	6.03 ± 1.54	6.67 ± 1.97	12.41 ± 3.08	46.35 ± 14.01	2.94 ± 0.99	3.25 ± 1.33	2.66 ± 1.08
19.48 ± 5.62	34.68 ± 10.24	7.75 ± 2.42	6.94 ± 2.11	13.82 ± 4.15	52.33 ± 16.85	3.67 ± 1.0	3.75 ± 1.79	4.04 ± 2.55
22.51 ± 5.49	40.13 ± 9.54	6.88 ± 1.62	7.35 ± 1.95	16.17 ± 3.81	77.09 ± 28.47	4.96 ± 1.67	4.64 ± 2.15	4.32 ± 2.13
24.14 ± 9.8	41.34 ± 14.93	9.26 ± 1.93	9.08 ± 1.78	17.28 ± 3.74	79.84 ± 24.17	5.17 ± 0.97	4.71 ± 2.02	5.94 ± 2.67
24.67 ± 6.75	48.65 ± 15.94	11.2 ± 3.59	10.44 ± 2.85	19.69 ± 6.14	72.82 ± 27.02	5.17 ± 1.62	6.4 ± 2.59	6.74 ± 3.7
25.87 ± 6.07	48.31 ± 11.72	10.26 ± 1.86	10.6 ± 1.9	20.99 ± 4.33	82.16 ± 25.54	5.97 ± 1.67	7.65 ± 3.08	7.09 ± 3.36
29.19 ± 6.34	52.5 ± 11.36	10.22 ± 3.22	10.77 ± 3.37	20.8 ± 5.12	93.25 ± 33.49	6.74 ± 2.48	6.8 ± 2.83	7.57 ± 3.58
29.98 ± 5.51	52.18 ± 10.87	11.6 ± 2.94	12.07 ± 3.21	20.62 ± 6.0	90.41 ± 31.17	7.07 ± 2.13	9.32 ± 3.58	7.75 ± 3.41
32.94 ± 8.31	56.48 ± 10.08	12.3 ± 1.39	13.29 ± 2.87	23.66 ± 4.62	104.67 ± 23.44	7.0 ± 1.95	9.09 ± 2.92	7.97 ± 2.17
31.78 ± 4.65	56.15 ± 9.52	11.6 ± 2.16	11.74 ± 2.6	24.92 ± 6.83	93.51 ± 26.58	7.28 ± 1.8	9.54 ± 2.96	7.26 ± 3.02
37.47 ± 3.43	67.62 ± 6.33	13.7 ± 2.4	14.86 ± 0.82	24.68 ± 4.9	124.92 ± 28.63	5.68 ± 2.38	12.47 ± 1.56	10.52 ± 5.74

Table 11 Postmortem body and organ weights for femur length in non-macerated fetuses (BWCH data)

Femur (cm)	Body weight (g)	Brain (g)	Heart (g)	Left lung (g)	Right lung (g)	Left kidney (g)	Right kidney (g)	Kidney combined (g)	Liver (g)	Adrenal combined (g)	Spleen (g)	Thymus (g)
0.8	14.9 ± 5.7	3.14 ± 1.52	0.12 ± 0.04	0.17 ± 0.09	0.21 ± 0.12	0.09 ± 0.07	0.09 ± 0.06	0.11 ± 0.05	0.97 ± 0.39	0.09 ± 0.05	Missing data[a]	Missing data[a]
1	23.1 ± 9.4	4.59 ± 2.11	0.23 ± 0.13	0.37 ± 0.18	0.42 ± 0.2	0.11 ± 0.09	0.16 ± 0.12	0.19 ± 0.1	1.41 ± 0.43	0.13 ± 0.1	0.66 ± 1.01	0.77 ± 1.25
1.2	33.4 ± 11.3	8.48 ± 3.87	0.27 ± 0.13	0.49 ± 0.23	0.6 ± 0.32	0.14 ± 0.06	0.14 ± 0.06	0.29 ± 0.14	2.08 ± 1.08	0.18 ± 0.08	0.05 ± 0.04	0.05 ± 0.03
1.4	46.7 ± 16.8	9.44 ± 4.0	0.33 ± 0.09	0.77 ± 0.31	0.87 ± 0.39	0.19 ± 0.09	0.2 ± 0.1	0.27 ± 0.14	2.18 ± 1.15	0.22 ± 0.11	0.04 ± 0.01	0.05 ± 0.03
1.6	59.9 ± 17.2	12.84 ± 4.46	0.45 ± 0.18	1.0 ± 0.44	1.17 ± 0.51	0.25 ± 0.12	0.24 ± 0.12	0.45 ± 0.18	3.2 ± 1.53	0.33 ± 0.15	0.07 ± 0.03	0.07 ± 0.04
1.8	83.5 ± 18.8	16.17 ± 1.95	0.53 ± 0.12	1.29 ± 0.55	1.56 ± 0.61	0.31 ± 0.12	0.32 ± 0.11	0.72 ± 0.25	4.26 ± 1.82	0.4 ± 0.21	0.07 ± 0.03	0.07 ± 0.03
2	94.8 ± 23.5	17.45 ± 4.03	0.61 ± 0.16	1.55 ± 0.58	1.83 ± 0.68	0.38 ± 0.13	0.38 ± 0.12	0.71 ± 0.26	4.98 ± 1.99	0.47 ± 0.16	0.1 ± 0.05	0.1 ± 0.04
2.2	126.5 ± 25.0	20.56 ± 4.12	0.84 ± 0.15	2.1 ± 0.55	2.49 ± 0.67	0.56 ± 0.19	0.56 ± 0.21	1.0 ± 0.08	7.15 ± 1.97	0.72 ± 0.23	0.13 ± 0.06	0.16 ± 0.05
2.4	156.8 ± 22.3	26.81 ± 4.58	1.04 ± 0.24	2.41 ± 0.67	2.82 ± 0.8	0.69 ± 0.24	0.67 ± 0.23	1.32 ± 0.39	8.42 ± 3.35	0.82 ± 0.33	0.16 ± 0.08	0.17 ± 0.08
2.6	179.9 ± 24.7	34.42 ± 11.08	1.3 ± 0.31	2.21 ± 0.73	2.73 ± 0.88	0.9 ± 0.23	0.9 ± 0.23	1.59 ± 0.46	10.28 ± 3.03	0.83 ± 0.34	0.22 ± 0.09	0.2 ± 0.1
2.8	214.3 ± 46.6	36.38 ± 6.6	1.45 ± 0.3	3.05 ± 0.86	3.72 ± 0.93	1.08 ± 0.28	1.05 ± 0.31	2.01 ± 0.54	11.83 ± 3.81	1.09 ± 0.45	0.25 ± 0.11	0.29 ± 0.13
3	255.3 ± 34.5	42.42 ± 5.4	1.82 ± 0.52	3.4 ± 1.51	4.18 ± 1.6	1.19 ± 0.37	1.22 ± 0.34	2.87 ± 0.67	16.41 ± 3.45	1.41 ± 0.39	0.35 ± 0.13	0.33 ± 0.14
3.2	288.2 ± 49.2	49.16 ± 9.5	2.0 ± 0.45	3.67 ± 1.14	4.59 ± 1.68	1.35 ± 0.4	1.4 ± 0.44	2.69 ± 0.63	16.5 ± 5.75	1.36 ± 0.48	0.39 ± 0.15	0.45 ± 0.21
3.4	352.8 ± 51.4	60.62 ± 10.18	2.49 ± 0.5	4.64 ± 1.52	5.76 ± 1.78	1.73 ± 0.38	1.76 ± 0.33	3.32 ± 1.0	19.71 ± 5.7	1.57 ± 0.68	0.51 ± 0.17	0.59 ± 0.25
3.6	401.5 ± 51.0	63.87 ± 9.09	2.64 ± 0.5	4.95 ± 1.64	6.11 ± 1.94	1.78 ± 0.41	1.79 ± 0.42	3.81 ± 0.93	21.66 ± 6.67	1.69 ± 0.61	0.61 ± 0.32	0.69 ± 0.29
3.8	430.2 ± 55.1	70.69 ± 8.68	3.08 ± 0.57	5.5 ± 1.67	6.66 ± 2.05	2.15 ± 0.67	2.14 ± 0.64	4.44 ± 1.36	25.58 ± 9.2	2.02 ± 0.88	0.59 ± 0.23	0.72 ± 0.3
4	499.4 ± 85.7	79.47 ± 14.07	3.31 ± 0.8	5.5 ± 1.56	6.65 ± 1.68	2.23 ± 0.82	2.15 ± 0.8	4.04 ± 0.99	23.09 ± 7.99	1.91 ± 0.57	0.68 ± 0.29	0.9 ± 0.44
4.2	602.5 ± 91.4	99.45 ± 17.58	4.03 ± 0.5	5.7 ± 1.25	7.44 ± 1.11	3.0 ± 1.04	3.04 ± 1.12	5.88 ± 2.13	27.23 ± 6.68	2.45 ± 1.07	0.91 ± 0.41	0.99 ± 0.46
4.4	677.6 ± 133.4	109.39 ± 27.71	4.21 ± 0.97	6.6 ± 1.67	8.13 ± 2.16	3.56 ± 1.07	3.33 ± 0.87	6.13 ± 1.85	31.36 ± 13.0	2.18 ± 0.74	1.15 ± 0.47	1.16 ± 0.51
4.6	721.4 ± 61.5	123.63 ± 14.47	4.39 ± 0.61	8.17 ± 2.07	9.74 ± 2.52	4.2 ± 2.1	4.27 ± 2.47	5.43 ± 1.44	29.22 ± 16.06	2.62 ± 0.73	0.96 ± 0.44	1.56 ± 1.09
4.8	771.0 ± 146.2	120.24 ± 21.79	4.76 ± 1.48	7.07 ± 1.83	8.56 ± 1.92	2.85 ± 0.78	2.64 ± 0.64	6.9 ± 2.54	29.36 ± 12.26	1.83 ± 0.65	1.45 ± 0.58	1.21 ± 0.56
5	996.9 ± 165.4	149.09 ± 21.01	6.53 ± 1.33	9.77 ± 2.3	11.96 ± 2.86	4.31 ± 1.99	4.46 ± 1.52	10.8 ± 2.57	44.61 ± 15.59	3.12 ± 1.33	2.32 ± 1.05	2.46 ± 1.13
5.2	1038.2 ± 218.2	155.93 ± 50.17	6.34 ± 1.67	10.48 ± 1.94	13.07 ± 2.16	5.05 ± 1.07	5.41 ± 1.2	9.91 ± 2.23	39.18 ± 12.92	2.8 ± 0.66	2.04 ± 0.9	2.19 ± 0.76
5.4	1255.1 ± 251.1	194.94 ± 51.73	9.97 ± 4.15	10.78 ± 5.62	12.97 ± 6.58	6.07 ± 0.46	6.47 ± 1.52	16.75 ± 9.84	54.74 ± 14.29	3.26 ± 1.73	5.12 ± 5.52	2.44 ± 1.38
5.6	1321.4 ± 249.5	196.53 ± 39.98	7.77 ± 2.37	11.73 ± 3.78	15.46 ± 5.17	6.26 ± 2.03	6.21 ± 1.86	12.16 ± 4.22	50.13 ± 22.15	3.6 ± 1.13	3.19 ± 1.86	2.59 ± 1.06

Table 11 (continued)

Femur (cm)	Body weight (g)	Brain (g)	Heart (g)	Left lung (g)	Right lung (g)	Left kidney (g)	Right kidney (g)	Kidney combined (g)	Liver(g)	Adrenal combined (g)	Spleen (g)	Thymus (g)
5.8	1335.8 ± 141.2	170.22 ± 55.45	7.78 ± 2.69	13.53 ± 5.05	16.16 ± 5.88	6.75 ± 0.35	7.3 ± 0.85	10.2 ± 4.51	51.13 ± 20.24	3.25 ± 1.12	3.38 ± 1.58	2.34 ± 1.66
6	1624.3 ± 253.1	247.96 ± 48.14	9.61 ± 1.84	15.16 ± 3.38	18.86 ± 4.39	8.22 ± 2.26	8.19 ± 2.37	13.92 ± 4.06	66.85 ± 23.2	4.1 ± 1.13	4.18 ± 1.56	3.87 ± 1.37
6.2	1795.4 ± 282.3	224.71 ± 27.97	10.53 ± 2.64	15.54 ± 4.1	19.8 ± 5.21	9.02 ± 2.91	9.53 ± 3.55	16.81 ± 7.34	72.91 ± 25.88	5.11 ± 1.8	5.42 ± 1.9	4.49 ± 2.57
6.4	1937.8 ± 248.1	265.11 ± 41.53	11.08 ± 2.71	18.2 ± 3.64	23.19 ± 5.1	8.98 ± 2.63	8.49 ± 2.41	16.74 ± 4.78	71.61 ± 24.29	4.37 ± 1.35	5.12 ± 1.9	5.4 ± 2.83
6.6	2159.3 ± 284.5	274.37 ± 47.96	13.75 ± 2.52	19.99 ± 4.03	24.57 ± 5.05	10.39 ± 2.96	12.82 ± 5.32	23.13 ± 5.96	85.52 ± 19.23	5.54 ± 1.51	6.15 ± 2.3	4.86 ± 2.36
6.8	2299.5 ± 322.9	299.32 ± 40.66	13.79 ± 2.84	21.13 ± 4.02	27.0 ± 4.73	10.63 ± 2.62	10.55 ± 2.53	19.83 ± 5.34	90.65 ± 29.62	6.46 ± 2.65	6.57 ± 2.56	6.58 ± 2.99
7	2603.8 ± 408.4	357.93 ± 20.98	17.13 ± 6.19	20.75 ± 3.0	25.42 ± 3.48	12.94 ± 5.79	12.68 ± 5.01	29.28 ± 8.75	98.57 ± 29.35	6.91 ± 2.55	6.51 ± 1.72	6.03 ± 2.18
7.2	2816.3 ± 347.4	362.08 ± 43.85	16.47 ± 2.95	23.34 ± 4.04	29.57 ± 4.85	12.33 ± 3.22	12.33 ± 3.85	23.13 ± 5.93	100.21 ± 27.6	6.89 ± 1.76	7.7 ± 2.66	8.2 ± 3.34
7.4	3051.0 ± 282.3	397.62 ± 43.83	16.55 ± 3.13	23.22 ± 3.72	30.32 ± 6.37	13.13 ± 2.73	12.72 ± 2.41	26.28 ± 2.31	118.41 ± 31.23	8.15 ± 2.99	8.74 ± 3.14	8.52 ± 2.75
7.6	3116.4 ± 327.0	395.78 ± 39.31	18.07 ± 3.0	27.32 ± 5.13	34.15 ± 7.34	14.47 ± 3.62	14.19 ± 3.5	26.51 ± 6.19	133.32 ± 38.57	8.71 ± 2.35	10.44 ± 3.73	10.58 ± 3.82
7.8	3371.9 ± 483.4	402.91 ± 35.7	20.11 ± 4.59	27.93 ± 6.21	35.9 ± 7.87	14.35 ± 2.39	15.41 ± 4.04	25.25 ± 3.53	147.31 ± 41.21	9.48 ± 2.33	10.69 ± 3.62	9.49 ± 3 05
8	3296.9 ± 381.3	408.75 ± 37.79	18.72 ± 3.06	27.99 ± 5.33	34.99 ± 6.62	15.34 ± 3.33	15.08 ± 3.0	26.49 ± 7.32	145.0 ± 40.52	9.22 ± 2.07	12.2 ± 3.83	9.82 ± 3.4
8.2	3573.2 ± 192.4	411.36 ± 21.86	19.88 ± 2.53	28.49 ± 4.85	35.95 ± 6.18	12.67 ± 3.29	13.9 ± 2.58	30.35 ± 4.49	157.59 ± 52.65	11.33 ± 2.91	11.02 ± 4.1	11.68 ± 4.79
8.4	3738.9 ± 408.0	420.08 ± 30.1	20.15 ± 3.34	31.71 ± 6.46	42.65 ± 10.79	15.34 ± 1.48	14.4 ± 1.98	24.94 ± 6.34	164.68 ± 48.4	9.55 ± 1.37	12.79 ± 3.62	10.92 ± 2.32

ᵃInsufficient number of valuables for analysis

Table 12 Postmortem body and organ weights for femur length in macerated fetuses (BWCH data)

Femur (cm)	Body weight (g)	Brain (g)	Heart (g)	Left lung (g)	Right lung (g)	Kidney combined (g)	Liver (g)	Adrenal combined (g)	Spleen (g)	Thymus (g)
0.8	14.9 ± 5.7	2.77 ± 1.59	0.14 ± 0.06	0.21 ± 0.09	0.25 ± 0.13	0.13 ± 0.07	0.86 ± 0.33	0.1 ± 0.05	Missing data[a]	Missing data[a]
1.0	20.5 ± 8.3	4.67 ± 2.23	0.16 ± 0.04	0.28 ± 0.12	0.33 ± 0.15	0.13 ± 0.06	0.99 ± 0.38	0.11 ± 0.06	Missing data[a]	Missing data[a]
1.2	26.9 ± 9.7	5.68 ± 2.15	0.23 ± 0.09	0.42 ± 0.23	0.51 ± 0.29	0.18 ± 0.09	1.49 ± 0.53	0.16 ± 0.07	0.04 ± 0.03	0.04 ± 0.02
1.4	33.8 ± 10.8	8.32 ± 4.91	0.27 ± 0.09	0.46 ± 0.14	0.55 ± 0.19	0.22 ± 0.08	1.66 ± 0.71	0.17 ± 0.06	0.04 ± 0.02	0.03 ± 0.01
1.6	48.1 ± 13.2	10.03 ± 3.52	0.35 ± 0.11	0.7 ± 0.27	0.86 ± 0.32	0.31 ± 0.11	2.21 ± 0.94	0.24 ± 0.09	0.06 ± 0.04	0.06 ± 0.03
1.8	68.8 ± 24.4	13.13 ± 5.53	0.45 ± 0.11	0.99 ± 0.35	1.22 ± 0.47	0.46 ± 0.16	2.69 ± 0.99	0.32 ± 0.11	0.08 ± 0.04	0.07 ± 0.04
2.0	79.5 ± 22.8	16.42 ± 4.74	0.56 ± 0.18	1.16 ± 0.54	1.38 ± 0.63	0.61 ± 0.33	3.0 ± 1.15	0.37 ± 0.12	0.08 ± 0.04	0.08 ± 0.04
2.2	103.6 ± 29.4	21.83 ± 6.84	0.68 ± 0.19	1.41 ± 0.4	1.64 ± 0.46	0.67 ± 0.33	3.53 ± 1.5	0.43 ± 0.15	0.09 ± 0.05	0.09 ± 0.04
2.4	124.4 ± 32.0	24.27 ± 6.55	0.8 ± 0.18	1.5 ± 0.44	1.84 ± 0.53	0.84 ± 0.38	3.91 ± 1.49	0.45 ± 0.12	0.15 ± 0.15	0.11 ± 0.06
2.6	141.3 ± 28.6	29.3 ± 8.38	0.88 ± 0.13	1.62 ± 0.71	1.95 ± 0.84	1.06 ± 0.41	5.24 ± 2.67	0.53 ± 0.2	0.16 ± 0.07	0.14 ± 0.07
2.8	185.3 ± 47.8	39.26 ± 10.39	1.21 ± 0.32	2.09 ± 0.86	2.52 ± 1.01	1.22 ± 0.37	6.46 ± 2.85	0.65 ± 0.22	0.19 ± 0.09	0.17 ± 0.08
3.0	222.5 ± 52.2	43.47 ± 11.98	1.45 ± 0.43	2.5 ± 1.1	2.99 ± 1.16	1.68 ± 0.54	7.64 ± 4.08	0.74 ± 0.26	0.22 ± 0.1	0.2 ± 0.09
3.2	265.9 ± 84.6	48.42 ± 14.68	1.73 ± 0.52	2.6 ± 0.82	3.28 ± 1.01	1.9 ± 0.58	9.89 ± 4.87	0.94 ± 0.4	0.34 ± 0.16	0.26 ± 0.14
3.4	298.8 ± 75.0	49.96 ± 18.93	1.91 ± 0.63	2.69 ± 0.8	3.08 ± 0.71	2.19 ± 0.4	8.95 ± 3.19	0.95 ± 0.43	0.35 ± 0.2	0.27 ± 0.14
3.6	327.5 ± 73.4	62.95 ± 13.7	2.21 ± 0.6	2.84 ± 0.7	3.66 ± 1.01	2.77 ± 0.83	11.95 ± 4.54	0.99 ± 0.29	0.37 ± 0.18	0.39 ± 0.21
3.8	378.5 ± 85.3	64.36 ± 17.42	2.49 ± 0.65	3.23 ± 0.98	4.32 ± 0.8	2.56 ± 0.48	11.06 ± 4.06	1.34 ± 0.45	0.42 ± 0.2	0.45 ± 0.2
4.0	441.5 ± 82.2	76.25 ± 16.99	2.82 ± 0.7	4.09 ± 1.09	5.17 ± 1.38	3.44 ± 1.25	14.99 ± 5.98	1.32 ± 0.54	0.62 ± 0.35	0.55 ± 0.26
4.2	490.9 ± 120.9	90.95 ± 6.84	3.27 ± 0.87	4.63 ± 1.94	5.88 ± 2.37	3.76 ± 1.07	15.54 ± 6.33	1.4 ± 0.49	0.68 ± 0.29	0.48 ± 0.2
4.4	680.9 ± 140.2	104.52 ± 27.08	3.85 ± 1.06	5.43 ± 1.4	6.77 ± 1.72	5.51 ± 1.67	21.37 ± 7.88	1.77 ± 0.41	1.16 ± 0.54	0.86 ± 0.35
4.6	814.3 ± 202.2	118.15 ± 26.18	6.38 ± 3.01	8.16 ± 2.21	9.03 ± 1.16	8.64 ± 2.18	29.04 ± 8.96	2.33 ± 0.67	1.07 ± 0.4	0.75 ± 0.7
4.8	817.7 ± 210.1	121.75 ± 33.57	5.6 ± 2.62	6.42 ± 1.62	8.6 ± 2.52	6.47 ± 2.62	27.64 ± 13.48	2.12 ± 0.8	1.69 ± 1.14	1.08 ± 0.5
5.0	924.0 ± 87.5	146.81 ± 30.49	5.13 ± 1.01	7.92 ± 2.2	9.77 ± 2.61	Missing data[a]	29.17 ± 13.11	2.51 ± 1.46	1.82 ± 1.02	1.56 ± 0.61
5.2	1074.1 ± 225.2	157.85 ± 29.74	6.15 ± 1.49	8.38 ± 1.7	10.32 ± 2.27	9.17 ± 2.71	34.2 ± 9.9	2.4 ± 0.59	1.95 ± 0.59	1.63 ± 0.58
5.4	1173.8 ± 176.2	160.87 ± 22.48	6.7 ± 1.74	10.12 ± 1.49	12.39 ± 2.15	8.27 ± 1.68	35.85 ± 11.35	2.27 ± 0.49	2.2 ± 0.9	2.29 ± 0.88
5.6	1269.5 ± 189.6	177.21 ± 23.58	7.56 ± 1.61	11.57 ± 2.94	14.65 ± 2.36	9.81 ± 2.81	39.08 ± 10.91	3.25 ± 1.1	2.27 ± 1.07	2.34 ± 0.92
5.8	1392.6 ± 191.6	188.49 ± 26.53	9.15 ± 3.97	11.63 ± 0.96	14.5 ± 1.49	8.65 ± 2.14	43.07 ± 9.3	3.39 ± 0.75	2.67 ± 1.48	1.93 ± 1.09
6.0	1574.7 ± 242.3	233.36 ± 50.15	9.88 ± 2.4	14.57 ± 4.01	17.61 ± 4.96	12.09 ± 2.39	48.56 ± 14.32	3.0 ± 1.03	4.06 ± 1.8	3.24 ± 1.22
6.2	1757.4 ± 243.6	250.41 ± 31.56	11.91 ± 3.21	11.9 ± 3.72	15.54 ± 4.0	17.1 ± 7.48	57.93 ± 18.26	3.59 ± 1.09	5.06 ± 1.77	2.09 ± 1.07

Table 12 (continued)

Femur (cm)	Body weight (g)	Brain (g)	Heart (g)	Left lung (g)	Right lung (g)	Kidney combined (g)	Liver (g)	Adrenal combined (g)	Spleen (g)	Thymus (g)
6.4	1960.3 ± 345.6	257.62 ± 41.91	12.53 ± 4.39	16.86 ± 5.14	21.48 ± 5.85	15.51 ± 3.25	58.18 ± 21.45	4.14 ± 1.06	3.91 ± 1.8	4.53 ± 2.27
6.6	2055.8 ± 204.3	293.03 ± 48.65	11.6 ± 2.03	16.66 ± 2.29	21.38 ± 4.04	17.3 ± 3.59	60.91 ± 12.57	4.81 ± 1.19	4.15 ± 1.65	5.22 ± 3.5
6.8	2333.0 ± 369.2	306.13 ± 36.56	13.71 ± 3.07	19.42 ± 4.82	24.74 ± 5.39	17.19 ± 4.52	73.27 ± 21.3	4.86 ± 1.48	5.59 ± 2.3	5.68 ± 2.4
7.0	2718.0 ± 370.0	350.87 ± 31.67	14.94 ± 3.56	24.45 ± 8.88	28.06 ± 8.06	19.88 ± 4.98	88.4 ± 24.13	6.86 ± 2.11	6.46 ± 2.12	5.58 ± 1.9
7.2	2834.0 ± 341.1	342.28 ± 41.77	16.6 ± 3.74	23.36 ± 4.44	29.34 ± 5.44	22.14 ± 5.38	91.47 ± 25.03	6.55 ± 1.58	7.29 ± 2.58	8.01 ± 2.6ᵃ
7.4	3016.3 ± 450.3	367.35 ± 36.08	16.66 ± 3.32	24.33 ± 3.86	29.92 ± 5.29	21.16 ± 4.1	84.62 ± 23.49	6.37 ± 1.79	8.02 ± 2.97	9.09 ± 3.1
7.6	3081.0 ± 393.4	371.73 ± 47.69	16.58 ± 3.64	24.25 ± 4.26	31.07 ± 5.71	23.36 ± 4.92	94.12 ± 28.83	6.93 ± 2.02	8.91 ± 3.3	8.06 ± 3.38
7.8	3365.2 ± 618.1	386.65 ± 50.5	19.64 ± 4.38	27.62 ± 9.38	33.56 ± 9.78	18.41 ± 1.58	111.36 ± 28.78	7.69 ± 2.01	12.85 ± 1.52	8.85 ± 2.68
8.0	3250.8 ± 394.0	412.27 ± 40.58	19 1 ± 5.56	25.49 ± 4.78	32.1 ± 5.89	24.74 ± 10.54	111.85 ± 19.71	7.33 ± 2.1	9.4 ± 3.03	8.9 ± 3.73
8.2	3982.7 ± 838.1	419.0 ± 17.35	23 94 ± 8.24	30.49 ± 8.51	37.32 ± 10.2	Missing dataᵃ	131.7 ± 22.19	7.91 ± 2.13	15.21 ± 6.28	7.52 ± 1.04
8.4	3352.0 ± 330.9	431.93 ± 37.77	16 66 ± 3.15	24.77 ± 6.36	31.66 ± 6.97	23.29 ± 6.2	99.41 ± 16.97	6.49 ± 1.86	9.17 ± 1.48	9.93 ± 2.16

ᵃInsufficient number of valuables for analysis

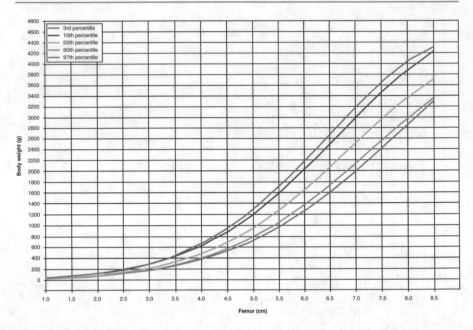

Fig. 4 Body weight curves for femur length in non-macerated fetuses (belongs to Table 11)

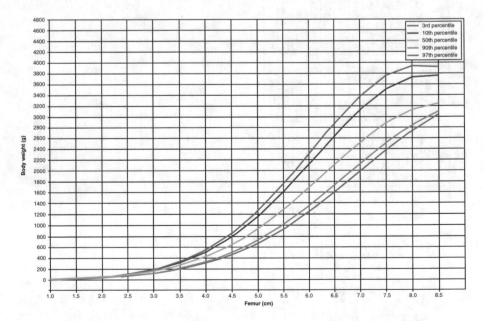

Fig. 5 Body weight curves for femur length in macerated fetuses (belongs to Table 12)

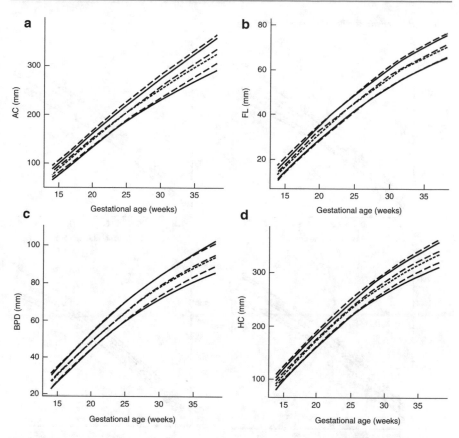

Fig. 6 DCDA Twin growth reference ranges. (From Stirrup, O. T., Khalil, A., D'Antonio, F., Thilaganathan, B. (2015), Fetal growth reference ranges in twin pregnancy: analysis of the Southwest Thames Obstetric Research Collaborative (STORK) multiple pregnancy cohort. Ultrasound ObstetGynecol, 45: 301–307. doi:https://doi.org/10.1002/uog.14640 with permission)

Fetal growth reference ranges in twin pregnancy

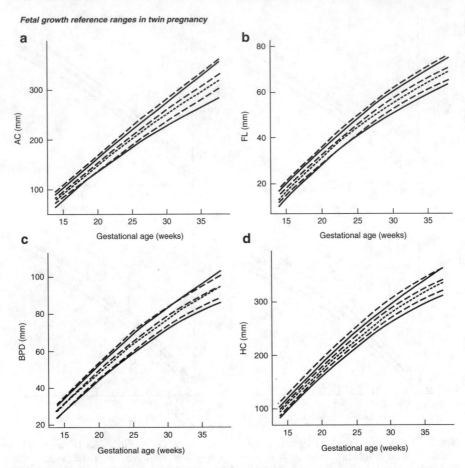

Fig. 7 MCDA Twin growth reference ranges. (From Stirrup, O. T., Khalil, A., D'Antonio, F., Thilaganathan, B. (2015), Fetal growth reference ranges in twin pregnancy: analysis of the Southwest Thames Obstetric Research Collaborative (STORK) multiple pregnancy cohort. Ultrasound ObstetGynecol, 45: 301–307. doi:https://doi.org/10.1002/uog.14640 with permission)

Calculating Organ to Organ Weight Ratios, Working with Computerized Charts and Calculators

When autopsy has been completed, careful analysis of the collected data has to follow, this is the stage when the case needs to be classified according to live birth or not, degree of maceration, singleton or multiple gestation, etc., and the appropriate reference charts have to be selected. In intrauterine death cases, gestational age needs to be adjusted considering the degree of maceration. In view of the ever-growing amounts of datasets and normal charts, it would be more comfortable and perhaps more standardized to use computer-based applications which are able to compare our data to the normal, calculate percentile, highlight abnormalities, and even perform calculations of organ ratios. A generous supply of standard tables, growth charts, publications, training recourses, and calculator applications—including centile calculator, gestational age calculator, expected fetal weight calculator—are available (free) at www.gestation.net/ [16] of the Perinatal Institute and at the website of the International Fetal and Newborn Growth Consortium for the 21st Century, or Intergrowth-21st at https://intergrowth21.tghn.org/ [17], recommended for clinicians but can be useful for perinatal pathologists as well.

A helpful autopsy calculator based on standard autopsy tables [2] is available at http://autopsy.jarchie.com which performs instant analysis of biometrical data saving time and effort. A novel software was developed to help the user to evaluate data faster and easier, highlight measurement and organ weight discrepancies, enabling users to identify abnormalities and to create more reliable report [18].

References

1. Muller Brochut AC, Taffe P, Piaget-Rossel R, de Leval L, Rougemont AL. Fetal Anthropometric features: a postmortem study of fetuses after the termination of pregnancy for psychosocial reasons between 12 and 20 gestational weeks. Pediatr Dev Pathol. 2019;22(3):243–51. https://doi.org/10.1177/1093526618812528. Epub 2018 Nov 19.
2. Archie JG, Collins JS, Lebel RR. Quantitative standards for fetal and neonatal autopsy. Am J Clin Pathol. 2006;126(2):256–65.
3. Merlob P, Sivan Y, Reisner SH. Anthropometric measurements of the newborn infant (27 to 41 gestational weeks). Birth Defects Orig Artic Ser. 1984;20(7):1–52.
4. Omotade O. Facial measurements in the newborn (towards syndrome delineation). J Med Genet. 1990;27:358–62. https://doi.org/10.1136/jmg.27.6.358.
5. Chitty LS, Altman DG. Charts of fetal size: limb bones. BJOG. 2002;109:919–29. https://doi.org/10.1111/j.1471-0528.2002.01022.x.
6. Gardosi J, Francis A, Turner S, Williams M. Customized growth charts: rationale, validation and clinical benefits. Am J Obstet Gynecol. 2018;218(2S):S609–18. https://doi.org/10.1016/j.ajog.2017.12.011.
7. Kiserud T, Benachi A, Hecher K, Perez RG, Carvalho J, Piaggio G, Platt LD. The World Health Organization fetal growth charts: concept, findings, interpretation, and application. Am J Obstet Gynecol. 2018;218(2S):S619–29. https://doi.org/10.1016/j.ajog.2017.12.010.
8. Villar J, Cheikh Ismail L, Victora CG, Ohuma EO, Bertino E, Altman DG, Lambert A, Papageorghiou AT, Carvalho M, Jaffer YA, Gravett MG, Purwar M, Frederick IO, Noble AJ, Pang R, Barros FC, Chumlea C, Bhutta ZA, Kennedy SH, International Fetal and Newborn Growth Consortium for the 21st Century (INTERGROWTH-21st). International standards for newborn weight, length, and head circumference by gestational age and sex: the Newborn Cross-Sectional Study of the INTERGROWTH-21st Project. Lancet. 2014;384(9946):857–68. https://doi.org/10.1016/S0140-6736(14)60932-6.
9. Khong TY. The perinatal necropsy. In: Khong TY, Malcomson RDG, editors. Keeling's fetal and neonatal pathology. 5th ed. London: Springer; 2015.
10. Pryce JW, Bamber AR, Ashworth MT, Kiho L, Malone M, Sebire NJ. Reference ranges for organ weights of infants at autopsy: results of >1,000 consecutive cases from a single centre. BMC Clin Pathol. 2014;14:18. https://doi.org/10.1186/1472-6890-14-18. eCollection 2014.
11. Scheimberg I, Ashal H, Kotiloglu-Karaa E, French P, Kay P, Cohen MC. Weight charts of infants dying of sudden infant death in England. Pediatr Dev Pathol. 2014;17(4):271–7. https://doi.org/10.2350/13-08-1362-OA.1. Epub 2014 May 23.
12. Maroun LL, Graem N. Autopsy standards of body parameters and fresh organ weights in

nonmacerated and macerated human fetuses. Pediatr Dev Pathol. 2005;8(2):204–17. Epub 2005 Mar 8.

13. Stirrup OT, Khalil A, D'Antonio F, Thilaganathan B. Fetal growth reference ranges in twin pregnancy: analysis of the Southwest Thames Obstetric Research Collaborative (STORK) multiple pregnancy cohort. Ultrasound Obstet Gynecol. 2015;45:301–7. https://doi.org/10.1002/uog.14640.

14. Thayyil S, Schievano S, Robertson NJ, Jones R, Chitty LS, Sebire NJ, Taylor AM, MaRIAS (Magnetic Resonance Imaging Autopsy Study) Collaborative Group. A semi-automated method for non-invasive internal organ weight estimation by post-mortem magnetic resonance imaging in fetuses, newborns and children. Eur J Radiol. 2009;72(2):321–6. https://doi.org/10.1016/j.ejrad.2008.07.013. Epub 2008 Sep 2.

15. Man J, Hutchinson JC, Ashworth M, Jeffrey I, Heazell AE, Sebire NJ. Organ weights and ratios for postmortem identification of fetal growth restriction: utility and confounding factors. Ultrasound Obstet Gynecol. 2016;48(5):585–90. https://doi.org/10.1002/uog.16017. Epub 2016 Oct 25.

16. Perinatal Institute @ www.gestation.net.

17. Publications, charts and training recourses of Intergrowth-21 @https://intergrowth21.tghn.org/.

18. Cain MD, Siebert JR, Iriabho E. Development of novel software to generate anthropometric norms at perinatal autopsy. Pediatr Dev Pathol. 2015;18:203–9.

Diagnostic Criteria of Fetal Growth Abnormalities and Interpretation of Postmortem Size and Weight Measurements

Beata Hargitai

Clinical and Pathological Diagnostic Criteria of Fetal Growth Abnormalities

Problems of fetal growth can be related to environmental conditions, pre-existing or pregnancy related medical conditions of the mother or can be genetically predisposed or determined. Placental "cause" is a popular historic misnomer as the pathology of the feto-maternal interface and the placenta is not the origin but the consequence of the underlying anomalies—systemic or localized disease of maternal vessels, aberrant immune (alloimmune) response to villous antigens, maternal viral infection, or thrombophilia.

A large for gestational age (LGA) baby grows steadily above the 90th percentile, a small for gestational age (SGA) baby falls below the 10th percentile. Numerical definition of "low birth weight" is 2500 g and cut-off value of fetal overgrowth is 4500 g.

A difference is emphasized between growth dynamic of fetal growth restriction (FGR) and SGA, when in FGR—instead of the gradual increase of weight but on a low centile—the fetal growth tails off reaching a plateau, remaining steady and the fetus will not reach its growth potential. A proportion of SGA, and even normally grown (appropriate for gestational age, AGA) babies falls under the umbrella of FGR.

In the course of antenatal monitoring, abnormal ultrasound and Doppler findings and maternal tests can raise suspect and confirm FGR. Huge significance is attached to importance of prenatal diagnosis of the condition since unrecognized fetal growth restriction proved to be the single largest avoidable risk factor of stillbirth [1].

B. Hargitai (✉)
West Midlands Perinatal Pathology, Birmingham Women's and Children's Hospital, Birmingham, UK
e-mail: Beata.Hargitai@nhs.net

© Springer Nature Switzerland AG 2021
J. Martinovic (ed.), *Practical Manual of Fetal Pathology*,
https://doi.org/10.1007/978-3-030-42492-3_6

A shrinking but still significant proportion of cases is diagnosed on postmortem examination and one of the useful diagnostic tools of perinatal pathologists include detailed analysis of biometrical data. Calculations of organ to organ weight ratios, often used by pathologists in everyday practice and bearing with impact on diagnostic work, include body weight to placenta weight ratio (BW/PW), lung to body weight ratio (L/B), brain to liver weight ratio (B/L), and brain to thymus weight ratio (B/Th). Increased BW/PW (~7 at term is normal; >9–10 is abnormal) is suggestive of placental insufficiency. L/B is widely used for diagnosis of pulmonary hypoplasia and can be diminished or indicate established hypoplasia in severe, prolonged growth restriction [2, 3]. Lower limit of normality is 0.012 above the 28th week of gestation, and 0.015 before 28th week of gestation [2]. Normal B/L (normal between 2–4 and 6 depending on maceration) is a recognized indicator of asymmetrical growth restriction and elevated B/Th is associated to significant and ongoing intrauterine stress (normal up to 50 at term).

Diagnostic criteria of various categories in growth abnormalities are far from being clear cut and definite. A commendable example to solve ambiguities is the Delphi protocol for clinical diagnosis of FGR, a collaboration between large, international group of obstetricians aiming to reach a consensus [4] and now the project is continuing with involvement of pathologists to create explicit pathological diagnostic criteria.

Interpretation of Postmortem Data

Importantly, the clinical context and the targeted questions of the postmortem examination always must be kept in the center. More often than not, the pathologist is faced with co-existing anomalies of measurements representing a mixture of artifacts and true pathology. Therefore, interpretation of findings lays with the investigating pathologist utilizing evidence-based information, judgement of observations, and personal experience. When interpreting fetal size and attempting to diagnose and classify growth abnormalities, in addition to measurements, weights, and ratios, results of other tests and examination have to be considered and amalgamated into the conclusion. For example, external observations of body proportions and macroscopic appearances or histological characteristics of the placenta can aid in diagnosis of asymmetrical growth restriction and in extreme case can suggest triploidy; or cherubic facial features in a large for date baby would raise suspect of maternal diabetes.

Based on current recommendations and suggestions of published references [5–8], the following practical guide, outlined in a flowchart format, can be helpful in everyday practice (Fig. 1). The flowchart attempts to demonstrate how information from clinical history, macroscopic findings, histological examination, and from genetic test results can be utilized, highlighting the role of biometrical measurements and their relations in the diagnostic pathway of fetal growth abnormalities. Far from being a rigid guideline, it may provide practical support for interpretation

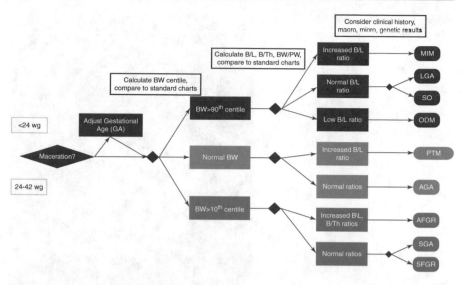

Fig. 1 Postmortem diagnostic patterns of fetal growth. *GA* gestational age, *BW* birth weight, *B/L* brain to liver weight ratio, *B/Th* brain to thymus weight ratio, *MIM* malnutrition in macrosomia, *LGA* large for gestational age, *SO* syndromic overgrowth, *ODM* overgrowth associated to maternal diabetes mellitus, *PTM* probable terminal malnutrition, *AGA* appropriate growth for age, *AFGR* asymmetrical fetal growth restriction, *SGA* small for gestational age, *SFGR* symmetrical fetal growth restriction. Color Codes: red—large for gestation based on birth weight centile >90%, grey—appropriate growth for age based on normal birth weight centile, blue—small for gestation based on birth weight centile <10%

of fetal biometrical data collected and calculated as a part of postmortem examination. Two classical examples (Figs. 2 and 3) are demonstrated below to illustrate the diagnostic steps which can be followed on the flowchart.

For evaluation of postmortem weight, the use of customized—or at least partially customized—birth weight centile is a recommended practice. Advantages of a local, or multi-ethnic population based standardized charts and centile calculators have been previously discussed. Conventional definition of appropriate growth is above the 10th and below the 90th (customized) centile.

In addition to comparing organ weights to the normal standard, calculation of organ to organ weight ratios can illuminate otherwise hidden growth anomaly—such as growth restriction in babies with appropriate weight for gestation—and may significantly modify the diagnostic route.

Brain to liver weight ratio is considered increased when exceeding 4 in non-macerated perinatal death cases and the cut-off criterion is over 6 in presence of moderate to severe maceration [5–8]. Significant fetal blood loss caused by ruptured vasa previa or feto-maternal transfusion leads to spurious increase of B/L, in contrast to severe congestion or chronic fetal anemia, when increased liver weight may lead to normal B/L in a growth restricted baby. Increased brain to thymus weight ratio (>50 from 32/40 weeks of gestation and >70 under 32/40 weeks gestation)

Fig. 2 Asymmetrical fetal growth restriction

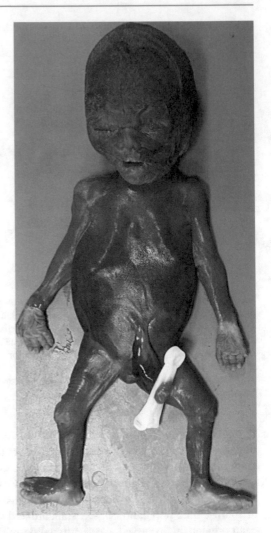

Example 1
Third trimester intrauterine death, diagnosed at 28/40 weeks gestation. Autopsy findings: Mild maceration, normal measurements for gestation, birth weight below the third customized centile, increased B/L ratio (5.9), increased B/Th ratio (122), lower weight for abdominal organs than expected, histology confirms chronic thymic stress, fatty changes of the adrenal cortex, and hypoxic-ischemic brain damage. The placenta weight is below the third centile, and histology shows chronic histiocytic intervillositis combined with massive perivillous fibrin deposition. Comment: This case is a classical example of asymmetrical fetal growth restriction caused by chronic placenta insufficiency due to underlying placenta pathology.

Fig. 3 Fetal overgrowth associated to maternal diabetes or pre-diabetes

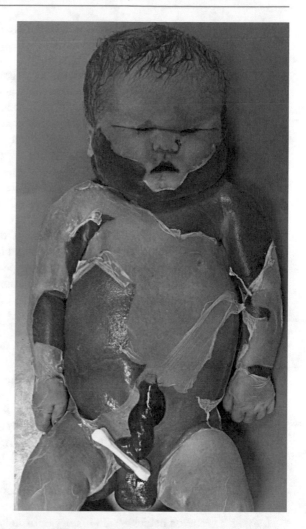

Example 2

IUD diagnosed at 38/40 weeks gestation, with history of decreased fetal movements and maternal obesity. Autopsy findings: Moderate maceration, infant with cherubic facial features and single umbilical artery. Birth weight falling on the 95th customized centile. Increased weight for the liver, low B/L weight ratio (1.8), normal B/Th weight ratio. Placenta weight just above the tenth centile, increased body weight to placenta weight ratio (9.3). Histology reveals hyperplasia of islets of Langerhans in the pancreas, villous edema, and high grade fetal vascular malperfusion in the placenta. Comment: This is a large for gestation baby and with additional clinical, macroscopic, and histological findings suggestive of fetal overgrowth associated to maternal diabetes or pre-diabetes (ODM).

with histology of chronic thymic stress is a supportive finding in fetal growth restriction, similarly to stress-related histological changes of the adrenal glands. Asymmetrical fetal growth restriction (AFGR) is associated to placenta insufficiency with histological evidence of chronic maternal vascular malperfusion, fetal vascular malperfusion, chronic alloimmune villitis and deciduitis, and chronic histiocytic intervillositis-massive perivillous fibrin deposition.

Symmetrical fetal growth restriction (SFGR) is characterized by general decrease of growth parameters including HC, with all organs equally affected, without the brain-spearing effect, unlike in AFGR, brain to liver weight ratio is normal, the thymus weight and other organ weight are lower than expected, the birth weight to placenta weight ratio can be normal or low. Examples, quoted by textbooks, include chromosomal abnormalities and viral infections—CMV or Rubella—, and in general, disorders which affect the embryo and fetus during the early stage of pregnancy, leading to loss of cell cycles and resulting in lower cell count.

Increased brain to liver weight ratio can be found in a population of fetuses and infants born with normal or higher weight than expected for gestational age. This finding can be regarded as indicator of nutritional and hypoxic stress, leading to significant nutritional impairment prior to death; interpreted in AGA babies as "probable terminal malnutrition (PTM)" and in LGA infants "malnutrition in macrosomia (MIM)." Brain to thymus weight ratio is usually increased and, especially in MIM, cherubic facial features and increased birth weight to placenta weight ratio can be seen as associated anomaly.

When the birth weight falls over the 90th centile and the brain to liver weight ratio is lower than 2, further indicators of maternal (gestational or pre-gestational) diabetes have to be investigated. Cherubic facial features, increased amount of subcutaneous fat, relatively large heart and lower brain weight are frequent associations, and hepatomegaly contributes to the low B/L ratio of babies with "overgrowth in context of maternal diabetes (ODM)." Even in absence of prenatal diagnosis, based on unequivocal postmortem findings underlying cause of maternal diabetes or pre-diabetes can be suggested, especially with history of increased maternal BMI.

Large for gestation babies—with history of usually unexpected stillbirth or sudden infant death—with normal organ to organ ratios, with or without evident-associated dysmorphic features, raise suspect of syndromic overgrowth and warrant for genetic testing and referral. Early death may occur in Beckwith–Wiedemann syndrome or in Sotos syndrome, and neonatal death is frequent in Perlman syndrome.

References

1. Gardosi J, Madurasinghe V, Williams M, Malik A, Francis A. Maternal and fetal risk factors for stillbirth: population based study. BMJ. 2013;346:f108.
2. Wigglesworth JS, Desai R, Guerrini P. Fetal lung hypoplasia: biochemical and structural variations and their possible significance. Arch Dis Child. 1981;56(8):606–15.

3. Laudy JA, Wladimiroff JW. The fetal lung. 2: pulmonary hypoplasia. Ultrasound Obstet Gynecol. 2000;16(5):182 94.
4. Gordijn SJ, Beune IM, Thilaganathan B, Papageorghiou A, Baschat A, Baker PN, Silver RM, Wynia K, Ganzevoort W. Consensus definition of fetal growth restriction: a Delphi procedure. Ultrasound Obstet Gynecol. 2016;48(3):333–9. https://doi.org/10.1002/uog.15884.
5. Marton T, Hargitai B, Bowen C, Cox PM. Elevated brain weight/liver weight ratio in normal body weight centile term perinatal deaths: an indicator of terminal intrauterine malnourishment. Pediatr Dev Pathol. 2013;16(4):267–71. https://doi.org/10.2350/12-11-1278-OA.1. Epub 2013 Apr 9.
6. Cox P, Marton T. Pathological assessment of intrauterine growth restriction. Best Pract Res Clin Obstet Gynaecol. 2009;23(6):751–64. https://doi.org/10.1016/j.bpobgyn.2009.06.006. Epub 2009 Oct 23.
7. Mitchell ML. Fetal brain to liver weight ratio as a measure of intrauterine growth retardation: analysis of 182 stillborn autopsies. Mod Pathol. 2001;14(1):14–9.
8. Man J, Hutchinson JC, Ashworth M, Jeffrey I, Heazell AE, Sebire NJ. Organ weights and ratios for postmortem identification of fetal growth restriction: utility and confounding factors. Ultrasound Obstet Gynecol. 2016;48(5):585–90. https://doi.org/10.1002/uog.16017. Epub 2016 Oct 25.

Part III

Fetal Autopsy

Abstract

Fetal autopsy is one of the essential approaches to perinatal care. In stillbirths, it contributes to determining the causes and timing of death. In medical terminations of pregnancy (TOP) regardless of fetal age, it serves as a quality control and assurance for fetal medicine, further refines the fetal phenotype, and directs molecular studies. Fetal autopsy results provide appropriate genetic counseling to parents and the management of future pregnancies for clinicians.

Preliminary Concerns to Enhance Fetal Examination Yield

Jelena Martinovic and Neil J. Sebire

In our era of genomic medicine embracing new horizons in fetal and perinatal pathology, novel terms have been introduced. The term "molecular autopsy" usually refers to the absence of feto-placental examinations and its replacement by prenatal biopsies for various genomic tests. While in some circumstances there may be a clear indication for a specific molecular genetic investigation, for accuracy it is suggested:

1. That the term "autopsy" should be reserved for phenotypic examinations (either complete or partial)
2. That molecular investigations should be included as a part of the modern fetal autopsy

Moreover, to confirm the clinical relevance of many unknown or rare variants of uncertain significance uncovered by genomic tests and to avoid false positive/negative conclusions, a dialogue is necessary concerning fetal phenotype with pathologists.

This manual provides the basic approach for the modern fetal autopsy which should be case-oriented rather than systematic in order to better serve patients by providing the most appropriate counseling possible.

Finally, despite increasing diagnostic yield from genomics in the prenatal setting (from 22% for various available next-generation sequencing (NGS) panels to over 50% for whole-genome sequencing (WGS)), the majority of fetuses will

J. Martinovic (✉)
Unit of Embryo-Fetal Pathology, University Hospitals AP-HP, Antoine Béclère,
Paris Saclay University, Clamart, France
e-mail: jelena.martinovic@aphp.fr

N. J. Sebire
Department of Histopathology, Great Ormond Street Hospital and ICH UCL, London, UK
e-mail: neil.sebire@gosh.nhs.uk

© Springer Nature Switzerland AG 2021
J. Martinovic (ed.), *Practical Manual of Fetal Pathology*,
https://doi.org/10.1007/978-3-030-42492-3_7

79

harbor a diagnosis apparent only from feto-placental examination, being linked to vascular, infectious, teratogenic, or multifactorial/complex causes yet to be elucidated.

Long live fetal pathology!

Indications for Fetal Autopsy

Every laboratory performing fetal exams should design its fetal autopsy referral criteria and request protocols very clearly in agreement with its clinical team. Naturally, the indication list may vary depending on ongoing clinical research programs or the level of prenatal care provided by the institution.

For example, in a tertiary care center for fetal medicine, the following indications have been established:

– In utero fetal demise (IUFD)
– Recurrent miscarriage (in index cases, placentas only)
– Medical terminations of pregnancy with normal FISH/karyotypes (or pending)
– In known aneuploidies, we acknowledge that the diagnosis has already been made by previous cytogenetic tests. Furthermore, in such cases, as TOPs for trisomy 21 for elevated first trimester markers and/or increased nuchal translucency, a fetal examination frequently remains silent and might not benefit the family.

Clinical Request

Every fetopathology laboratory should provide a concise request form with essentials for clinical autopsy or placental examination only, including an indication in the clinical context. A model for such a document is provided (Fig. 1). (1) The name and contact details of the clinician in charge; (2) the date and time of the delivery; (3) gestational age; (4) indication; (5) the mother's medical and obstetrical history; (6) the father's age and medical history; (7) mother's serologies; (8) fetal karyotype and micro-array; (9) any medication during the pregnancy or any other potentially teratogenic exposure; (10) copies of performed sonographic scans, eventually MRI and all other reports, and naturally any observation that the clinical staff deem relevant should be mentioned. Some institutions may provide computerized delivery reports as well.

For the fetuses from the same facility's maternity, the obstetric history might already be known. Causes may be thoroughly discussed during regular weekly prenatal multidisciplinary meetings, enabling the maximum amount of information to be collected in advance, as well as an optimal approach to examination and samplings.

CLINICAL QUESTIONNAIRE FOR FETO-PLACENTAL EXAMINATION	
FŒTUS & PLACENTA ☐	FŒTUS only ☐

ORDERING PHYSICIAN: .... INSTITUTION : ....

Contact phone #: ....

MOTHER's name: ....

First day of last period: ..../.............../.........

Date of pregnancy : ..../.............../.........

Date of TOP: ..../.............../.........

Date of expulsion : ..../.............../......... Hour :.....h.....

Date form completed :..............................

ID # (mother)

BABY (first name) : ....

Birth weight : .... g

Gender : .... Age : ....GW

INDICATION (TOP, IUFD, spontaneous abortion)

....
....
....

MOTHER	FATHER
Date of Birth:	Last name : ....
Medical history :	First name : ....
- personal :	Date of Birth : ....
- family :	Medical history :
- past pregnancies:	- personal : ....
....	....
....	....
....	
- gynaecological (contraception, infertility...) :	- family: ....
....	....
....	....
....	
Blood group : .... Ethnie:	Blood group : .... Ethnie : ....
Consanguinity : Yes☐ No ☐ Incertain ☐	

Fig. 1 Model of clinical form for fetal examination

ACTUAL PREGNANCY FOLLOW-UP

Maternal serologies :

HIV	HBS	HbC	Rubella	Toxoplasmosis Gondii
positive / negative / pending	positive / negative / pending	positive / negative / pending	positive/ negative / pending	positive/ negative / pending

Weight gain : ....kg

	1st Trimester	2nd Trimester	3rd Trimester
Medication (incl. over the counter) : Reason: Dose : Frequency :			
Smoking/ Alcohol			
Particular pathologies : High Blood Pressure / Diabetes / Anemia / Allergies / Infections / Metrorrhagia/ Fœto-maternal incomp./ Thrombophilia…			
US scans : (join copies)			

DELIVERY

Mode of delivery: ……………………………….   Duration: …………………………………...

Pathologies: ……………………………………………………………………………………………..

Duration of ruptured membranes: …………………………….   AF: ……………….

Hyperthermia: ……………………………………

Delivery (normal, hemorrhagic, artificial) : ……………………………………………………………………………….

REALIZED EXAMS

Bacteriological: …………………………………………………………………………………………

Karyotype: ………………………………………………………………………………………………..

Kleihauer test: ……………………………………………………………………

ADDITIONAL REMARKS

Join copies of all documents / results

Fig. 1 (continued)

Fetal Autopsy Consent

Although the consent for autopsy and its various ethical considerations are principally discussed in the first chapter of the manual, as a requirement "sine qua non" for fetal postmortem, regardless of age, a few additional points are briefly mentioned here.

The clinical team will offer the possibility of autopsy with appropriate parental consent in selected indications (discussed above). In this process, before making their final decision, a concise leaflet might be helpful to the family.

Written by the pathology staff, a fetopathology information leaflet offers overall information about the hospital postmortem examination and how it might provide value for the parents in the future. In addition to these general issues, such information should specify the individual procedure for each hospital/laboratory considering the various aspects of an autopsy procedure (timing, mortuary organization concerning cremation, burial or donation, opening hours, available photos, etc.). The parents may wish to understand the practical aspects of the examination, particularly regarding the preservation of fetal body integrity, viewing their baby before or after, and funeral arrangements. The principal medical terms that the parents are likely to meet in the autopsy procedure or in pathologic reports are explained in clear language. The range of different options: full, limited, external only (with/without X-rays or virtual imaging) postmortem examinations should be explained, including their respective advantages and disadvantages. The importance of obtaining diagnostic and/or research samples should also be explained, since many parents may be unaware of ongoing clinical research. Appropriate time spent discussing informed consent initially is of value since it is often particularly difficult to obtain retrospective consent for inclusion in studies.

For many parents, fetal autopsy still remains taboo. Everything that can help them better understand this issue may result in an increase in overall consent agreements.

It should be recognized that, while the final decision belongs to the mother or parents, the way that the clinician presents the procedure is important. To improve appropriate autopsy consent rates, a multidisciplinary approach is advisable which includes both prenatal meetings on a regular basis with systematic discussions of all future fetal patients, and clinico-pathologic correlations with feedback from the pathologists. The training of junior doctors in the obstetric team by a one- or few days' immersion in a fetopathologic laboratory is suggested. This is to defuse prejudices about fetal body dissection, regardless of religion or culture. Only a hand-to-hand approach among clinicians and pathologists with a high mutual level of respect may result in the parents' understanding and lead to an increase in consent agreements.

In general, several options are available for parents:

- *Full postmortem* (consent allowing the pathologist to choose the best approach for diagnosis)
- *Limited postmortem* (specifying body parts or organs authorized for examination)
- *External only* (photographs, X-rays/MRI) with/without biopsies)

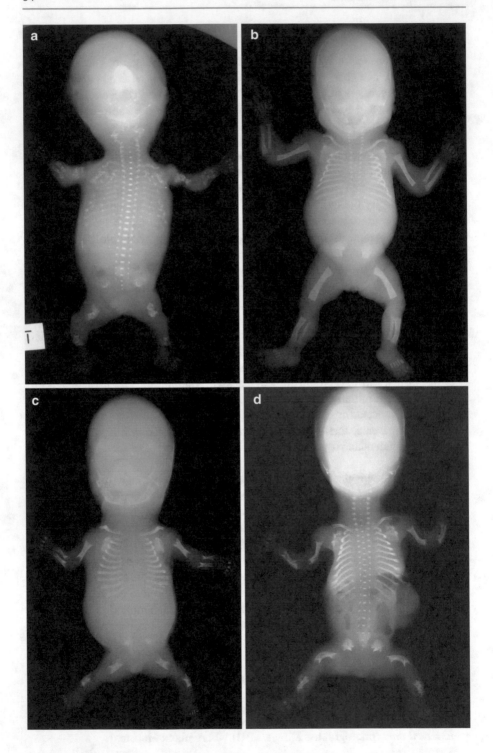

- Fetal biometry and external anomalies including facial appearance are performed in addition to radiologic fetal phenotype. Biopsies might be taken for targeted studies, including molecular or genomic evaluation.
- *No postmortem examination*
- Absence of any examination (radiologic/external/internal), and no physical or tissue archives, removing the possibility of any future evaluation which may be relevant in the case of recurrence.

The parents should also be informed that in some circumstances, if the diagnosis has already been determined by X-rays, external examination etc., even though they agreed to consent to full autopsy, the examination might be limited. In such cases, for example skeletal dysplasias, only local, i.e., knee cutaneo-muscular biopsies for DNA/molecular studies, and lower femoral fragment sampling for histology/chondrocyte cultures, might be sufficient (Fig. 2).

Fig. 2 Frontal whole body radiograms in first trimester fetuses terminated for the same clinical indication: "shortened long bones." Osteogenesis imperfecta (**a**); Hypochondrogenesis phenotype due to pathogenic variant (c.3121 G>A) in *COL2A1* (**b**); Achondrogenesis type II phenotype due to heterozygous de novo pathogenic variant (c.2663 G>A) in *COL2A1* (**c**). Thanatophoric dysplasia due to de novo *FGFR3* mutation (**d**)

Modern Fetal Autopsy Protocol

Jelena Martinovic and Neil J. Sebire

The six constituent parts of a full fetal postmortem examination are as follows:

1. Photographs
2. Fetal biometry
3. Fetal radiology
4. External clinical examination and phenotype analysis
5. Internal examination (gross/histology)
6. Fetal neuropathology

The first three procedures might be delegated, in their pre-analytic stage, to trained fetopathology technicians.

Only the principal procedures and their roles in performing fetal pathologic examination are described here: covering all aspects and in depth is beyond the scope of this manual.

Part 1: Photographs

Most fetal postmortems are performed in the fresh (unfixed) state following the fetal body being sent to the mortuary. It is important to systematically document findings through a series of external photographs, as well as of all abnormal findings during the autopsy procedure. A specialist macroscopy equipped camera is highly

J. Martinovic (✉)
Unit of Embryo-Fetal Pathology, University Hospitals AP-HP, Antoine Béclère,
Paris Saclay University, Clamart, France
e-mail: jelena.martinovic@aphp.fr

N. J. Sebire
Department of Histopathology, Great Ormond Street Hospital and ICH UCL, London, UK
e-mail: neil.sebire@gosh.nhs.uk

© Springer Nature Switzerland AG 2021
J. Martinovic (ed.), *Practical Manual of Fetal Pathology*,
https://doi.org/10.1007/978-3-030-42492-3_8

recommended. The camera distance from the stand should be constant allowing precise measurements of various anthropometric/cephalometric distances. A number of computer approaches are available to automatically archive the images in patient's (preferentially the mother's) records.

Pre-analytic, external standard photographs, performed in the laboratory by skilled technical staff, include:

1. One photo for parents/family (dressed as the fetus arrives, eventually with belongings, or covered properly for very macerated fetuses), with wristband identification
2. Whole body : anterior (front) view
3. Whole body: back view
4. Whole body : side views
5. Head : frontal view
6. Head: right and left profiles
   NB: Particular care should be taken to assuring correct profiles: one should follow the profile line entirely including fronto-nasal angle, columella, subnasion (philtrum), and menton (gnathion). In addition, the helix frequently covers the external meatus (positional effect), and thus auricle should be replaced correctly before taking pictures.
7. Hands and feet : close-up views

This eight-photo series may be expanded additionally for any unusual findings. In very small fetuses, with difficult to evaluate external genitalia, we suggest recording another specific photo of both external genitalia and perineum.

In some instances, i.e., special family request, the photo of the whole fetal body might be taken after an autopsy to clearly document body integrity.

Since parents may contact the hospital and request the photos of their baby several years after an examination, systematic archiving of the photos for families in patients' (mother's) records facilitates compliance with this request, and helps to improve the patients' relationship with medical providers.

Part 2: Fetal Biometry

External body measurements including body weight and length, vertex-coccyx distance, head circumference, and foot length before 29 weeks are biometric parameters for estimating fetal age. In our facility, they are systematically measured before an autopsy by trained and dedicated technicians.

It is worthwhile mentioning that while both imperial and metric systems are used for measurements, the metric system is preferred to standardize clinical fetopathologic reports worldwide.

Once fetal biometric measures are recorded, they should be compared to age-matched tables (see Part II). For non-macerated fetuses, these should be in agreement with expected fetal gestational age. Macerated fetuses, however, show various degrees of shift from the mean, which should be considered in fetal radiology and

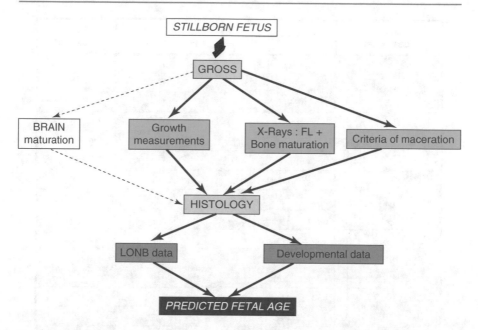

Fig. 1 Algorithm for predicting fetal age. In stillborn fetuses only combined: gross, histologic, and radiologic data may best predict the fetal age. *FL* femoral length, *LONB* loss of nuclear basophilia

biometry interpretation. Only assembly of all available predictive data: external biometry, radiology, and histology (skin, kidney, brain) offers an accurate estimate of in utero fetal retention and consequently fetal age (Fig. 1).

Part 3: Fetal Radiology

X-Ray

Fetal radiographs using plain X-ray are an integral part of the standardized fetal postmortem protocol. They are systematically performed and analyzed before external and internal examinations at any fetal age. It is highly advisable that each feto-placental pathology unit has a Faxitron and an image acquisition station, enabling each institution to maintain its own digitalized archives. In addition, there is a clear advantage to performing fetal radiographs by experienced, specialized staff. Three standard views for each fetus include: frontal whole body, limbs (in the same fetal position), and a whole body profile. Exposure time and power in kilovolts are defined for each gestational age from 14 to 41 weeks (Fig. 2).

Each fetopathologic team should determine their protocol for the number of systematic radiographs such as whole body for in utero fetal demises (IUFDs) or miscarriages (SAs), and additional imaging for complex, TOP cases. If a Faxitron is available, performing any additional radiographs is feasible if indicated.

Age (in gest. weeks)	Radiography type	Exposition time (in seconds)	Power (in kilovolts)
14	Extremities	10	20
	Face	20	30
	Profil	20	30
15	Extremities	10	25
	Face	20	35
	Profil	20	35
16	Extremities	11	25
	Face	22	35
	Profil	22	35
17	Extremities	11	27
	Face	22	37
	Profil	22	37
18	Extremities	12	25
	Face	25	35
	Profil	25	37
19	Extremities	12	27
	Face	25	37
	Profil	25	38
20	Extremities	15	22
	Face	30	32
	Profil	30	32
21	Extremities	15	23
	Face	30	33
	Profil	30	33
22	Extremities	15	25
	Face	30	35
	Profil	30	38
23	Extremities	15	31
	Face	30	41
	Profil	30	41
24	Extremities	15	33
	Face	30	43
	Profil	30	43

Fig. 2 Fetal radiologic values for Faxitron imaging (time of exposure in seconds, and power in kilovolts) for fetal age 14–41 weeks in different views/types (whole/face; hands/feet; whole profile)

Age (In gest. weeks)	Radiography type	Exposition time (in seconds)	Power (in kilovolts)
25	Extremities	15	35
	Face	30	45
	Profil	30	45
26	Extremities	15	37
	Face	30	47
	Profil	30	47
27	Extremities	20	35
	Face	40	45
	Profil	40	49
28	Extremities	25	40
	Face	50	50
	Profil	50	52
29	Extremities	20	45
	Face	40	55
	Profil	40	57
30	Extremities	30	45
	Face	60	55
	Profil	60	57
31	Extremities	45	47
	Face	90	57
	Profil	90	59
32	Extremities	45	48
	Face	90	58
	Profil	90	59
33	Extremities	50	44
	Face	100	54
	Profil	100	57
34	Extremities	55	45
	Face	110	55
	Profil	110	58
35	Extremities	60	44
	Face	120	54
	Profil	120	57

Fig. 2 (continued)

Age (in gest. weeks)	Radiography type	Exposition time (in seconds)	Power (in kilovolts)
36	Extremities	60	45
	Face	120	55
	Profil	120	58
37	Extremities	75	48
	Face	150	58
	Profil	150	60
38	Extremities	75	50
	Face	150	60
	Profil	150	62
39	Extremities	75	52
	Face	150	62
	Profil	150	64
40	Extremities	90	36
	Face	180	56
	Profil	180	60
41	Extremities	90	40
	Face	180	60
	Profil	180	70

Fig .2 (continued)

X-rays may also be used after injection studies with contrast in cases of sus-pected obstructing malformations as in urethral or tracheo-laryngeal stenosis versus atresias. Fine micro-probes frequently create iatrogenic perforations in small fetuses, thus careful intravesical/ intratracheal injections would allow assessment of luminal continuity before any further dissection.

In addition to femoral length, each developing fetus has its own bone maturation criteria. This information may be valuable for determining the precise fetal age (Fig. 3). Only key features for each gestational age are mentioned here. More detailed descriptions are available in the existing literature [1].

At 16 weeks, the vertebral bodies are visible from the C3-S3 level, and the iliac bones are square (Fig. 3a).

At 17 weeks, ischial bones become visible, superior ulnar metaphyses are con-vex, and second phalanges of fingers are square, except for the fifth fingers, where they are still round.

At 23 weeks, there is complete ossification of vertebral bodies to S4, ischio are vertical, and pubic bones become visible. The calcaneum is present.

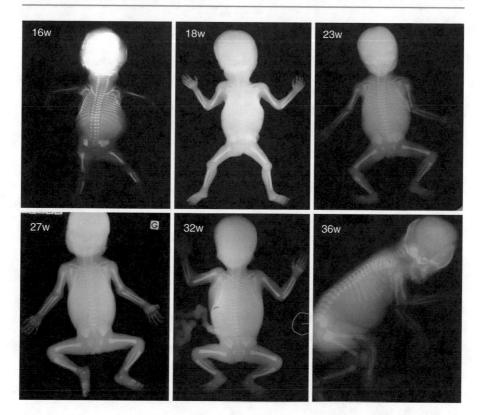

Fig. 3 Physiologic evolution in bone maturation of different ages from 16 to 36 weeks

At 27 weeks, sacrum is entirely ossified (S5), ischial bones are concave, and pubic bones are well developed. In addition to calcaneus, astragalus is present as well.

At 32 weeks, there are sharp margins of pubic bones, calcaneus and astragalus are well developed.

At 36 weeks, the distal femoral ossification epiphysis (Beclard) is always visible and proximal tibial ossification epiphysis (Todt) might be apparent as well. The sternum is visible, and the coccyx is entirely ossified.

These criteria allow an accurate evaluation of bone maturation and age. Advanced bone maturation may be observed in aneuploïdies.

For an interpretation of various skeletal anomalies, as well as their molecular backgrounds readers are advised to consult the published textbooks in which fetal skeletal anomalies are covered extensively [2]. Expert knowledge in fetal radiology is important to adequately direct fetal autopsies. In chondrodysplasia settings, identifying the disease already by pre-autopsy X-ray may, despite full postmortem consent, reasonably simplify and orient an autopsy to molecular biopsies and bone histologies.

MRI

Virtual fetal autopsy by magnetic resonance imaging (MRI) represents an option if the parents decline invasive fetal autopsy and for specific indications, which may be accompanied by tissue biopsies as appropriate.

Postmortem cross-sectional imaging is becoming established as a useful ancillary method either as a substitute for fetal dissection in cases where invasive autopsy is refused or as a part of the overall postmortem examination [3].

Part 4: External Examination/Fetal Phenotype

Phenotype, according to its current definition, represents an ensemble of physical and behavioral traits of the organism, resulting from the interaction of its genotype with the environment.

While the human phenome project [4] is still in the launch phase, current advances in DNA sequencing technologies and computational methods allow collecting of human phenotype data. It is therefore essential to employ precise and standard semantic terminology. The Human Phenotype Ontology has already more than 10,000 terms describing phenotypic anomalies in humans [5].

Despite quicker diagnoses via exome and genome sequencing in the future, there will remain challenges to understanding diseases through precise phenotyping [6]. Precise phenotypic descriptions allow: (1) stratifying patients into subpopulations, (2) establishing genotype/phenotype correlations, and (3) better understanding of the natural history of disease.

External fetal examinations should be assessed in the same manner as any other clinical genetic examination, however with identification of distinctive physiological signs specific for each age of a developing fetus. It is essential to be guided by these principles in order to avoid unnecessary and confusing false-positive results.

While different parts of the external examination may be performed simultaneously, we present them separately for didactic purposes.

Evaluation of the Degree of Maceration

Several studies on stillborn infants have determined how accurately the time of fetal death can be predicted from the extent of external maceration. Based on retrospective autopsy photographs of 86 stillborns with known time of death, eight gross features correlated reasonably well with specific death-to-delivery times in terms of sensitivity, specificity, and positive predictive values [7] including in increasing time interval order: desquamated skin measuring 1 cm or more in diameter and/or cord discoloration to brown/red (6 h); desquamation involving the skin of multiple body zones: face, back, or abdomen(12 h); desquamation of 5% or more of the body surface (18 h); brown or tan discoloration of the skin, usually involving the abdomen (24 h), and any mummification (2 weeks).

Others have suggested five stages of maceration [8, 9]:

1. None = intrapartum death
2. Slight—skin slippage, rare bullae, little (e.g., scrotum only or single spots of skin loss elsewhere) or no denudation = less than 12 h between death and delivery
3. Mild—focal denudation of multiple regions without other changes = about 12–24 h between death and delivery
4. Moderate—generalized skin maceration/denudation but without significant compressive changes = one to a few days between death and delivery
5. Advanced—compression and/or mummification and/or internal liquefaction = more than a few days between death and delivery

For practical reasons, we think that a simple staging system such as none, slight, moderate, and advanced maceration is generally sufficient. Along with other parameters of fetal maturation (radiologic and histologic), these may allow fine prediction of in utero retention time.

Overall Habitus

General fetal habitus should be carefully observed for:

- Color and appearance of fetal skin
- Body proportions
- In some cases, in addition to dwarfism, fetal growth might be disproportionate, i.e., for upper limbs or even hands. Since these measurements are not routinely included in pre-analytic fetal biometry, it is important not to overlook them at this stage of examination.
- Fingers and toes for their position, length, and any anomaly.
- Signs of in utero hypomobility expressed by distal or generalized contractures.

Importantly, any finding should always be correlated with fetal prenatal data. A lack of amniotic fluid by prematurely ruptured membranes can cause the anhydramnios (Potter) sequence which should not be mistaken or described as arthrogryposis, the latter term being reserved for intrinsic fetal neuro-muscular disorders. In the context of ruptured membranes, the terms articular deformities and oligo/anhydramnios sequence would be more appropriate.

Any prenatally diagnosed or newly identified observed anomaly should be systematically and precisely measured and documented photographically.

Clinical Dysmorphologic Evaluation

Fetal dysmorphological study is an essential, albeit complex, part of every feto-pathologic examination, fetal morphology evolving considerably with the age. Systematic examination of global fetal impression, i.e., gestalt, is needed,

combining standardized terminology (available at http://elementsofmorphology.
nih.gov/) and qualitative/descriptive terms. However, inter-observer impressions on
fetal dysmorphology varying considerably, pathologic terms should be introduced
only after comparison of each measurement with an age-related norm. Additionally,
facial measurements should be evaluated in regard to head circumference, since for
example normal outer canthal distance for age, in microcephalic fetuses means relative hypertelorism.

The hallmarks for evaluation of fetal cranio-facial dysmorphy, measured by
calipers, are presented together with the sources for normal values upon gestational age:

1. Occipito-frontal diameter (Normal values 12–41w from Hansmann 1985) [10]
2. Inner canthal distance (Normal values 27–41w from Merlob et al. 1984) [11]
3. Outer canthal distance (Normal values 27–41w from Merlob et al. 1984) [11]
4. Palpebral fissure length (Normal values 27–41w from Mehes et al. 1974) [12]
5. Philtrum length (Normal values 27–41w from Merlob et al. 1984) [11]
6. Mouth width/Intercommissural distance (Normal values from Merlob et al.
   1984) [11]
7. Ear length (Normal values 27–41w from Merlob et al. 1984) [11]

Textbooks are available [13] for further anthropometric measurements.

The goal of dysmorphology evaluation in fetuses is to recognize undiagnosed
syndromes and to consequently direct the rest of the fetal examination. Although
this is certainly feasible in older fetuses, the task remains difficult in first-trimester
terminations, expressing milder facial traits. Moreover, particular attention should
be paid to parents' ethnic backgrounds and general parents' phenotype. In that context, one should always privilege recording systematically facial measurements and
describing, rather than employing straightforward dysmorphology terminology
without anthropometric measurements (Fig. 4).

Part 5: Dissection/Internal Examination

Generally, dissection begins by the sharp median inverted Y-shaped incision
from the level of the thyroid or sternal notch, bypassing the umbilicus, towards
both inguinal regions. This is followed by separating the thoraco-abdominal skin
on each side. The pelvic triangle is dissected with blunt scissors to clearly visualize the urinary bladder and umbilical arteries. The thoracic cavity is opened by
vertically dissecting rib cartilages from diaphragmatic attachments on both sides
upwards, as laterally as possible, to the clavicles, removing median sterno-costal
fragment. An exception to this rule represents congenital diaphragmatic hernia/
eventrations, where the 12th rib with diaphragmatic attachment should be kept
intact, to allow better clinico-radiologic correlations, with precise descriptions,
measurements, and classification of an untouched diaphragmatic anomaly
(Fig. 5).

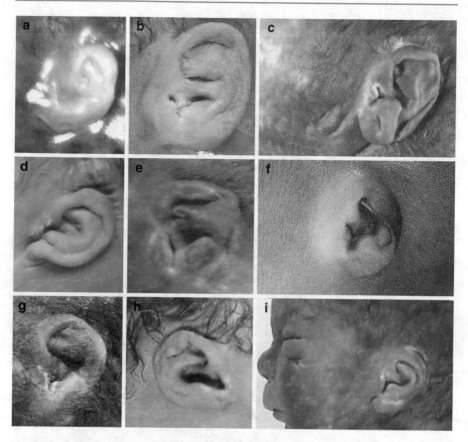

Fig. 4 Fetal ears: (**a**) Microtia in Treacher-Collins syndrome. (**b**) Normal fetal ear at 30w. (**c**) Wiedemann–Beckwith syndrome due to a methylation loss at ICR2 at 28w. (**d**) Trisomy 21 with horizontal crux helicis and rounded ears. (**e**) CHARGE syndrome due to *CHD7* variant. (**f**) Fryns syndrome. (**g**) Trisomy 18. (**h**) Di George syndrome due to 22q11 microdeletion. (**i**) Cornelia de Lange syndrome showing characteristic profile with hypoplastic ear, prominent philtrum, and unusually long eye lashes

In very small fetuses (13–16w) an inverted M-shaped incision (Fig. 6) may be preferred, meaning that secondary to the initial abdominal inverted V incision from the umbilicus, there are common, vertical costo-myo-cutaneous incisions on each side from the inguinal regions up to the clavicles, allowing easier opening by the elevation of a unique flap. In addition, reconstruction after an examination is simpler by turning the whole flap down.

In situ examinations and photographs for any observed anomaly are indicated. The thymus is removed first, and then weighed. Thymus and lung microbiopsies are routinely taken for tissue samples/DNA banking.

The pericardium should be completely removed on both sides to allow clear visualization of pulmonary vessels. Great vessels should be separated from each other from their base, and efferent aortic arteries dissected. Aortic arch, ductus

Fig. 5 Thoraco-abdominal opening variant in CDHs: last ribs with diaphragmatic attachment are kept intact

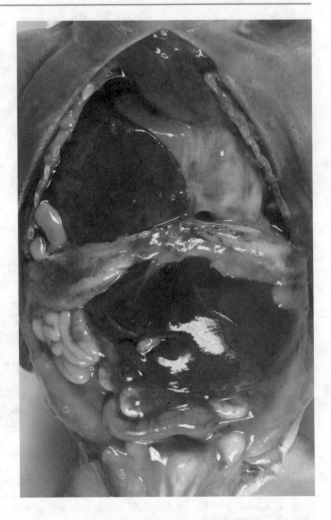

arteriosus, and descending aorta are checked for diameters and position. Ductus arteriosus diameter should be about the same as the preductal part of aortic arch throughout the pregnancy. This notion is important in assessing preductal aortic arch hypoplasias evolving towards coarctation. Before opening, the heart is inspected in situ. In addition to its vasculature, the position of anterior descending coronary arteries indicates ventricular size, and its shift to the right/left or its unusually short path signifies a hypoplastic or univentricular heart.

Opening of the heart follows the blood flow, and should be performed by sequential segmental analysis [14, 15] (Fig. 7).

We recommend dissecting all heart malformations fresh and directly on the photographic stand in order to record all aspects of heart opening from the in situ view to its left ventricular outflow. This might also help later clinico-pathologic correlations with ultrasound expertise on CHDs. Micro instruments, and a magnifying glass may be necessary for the dissection of first-trimester hearts (Fig. 8).

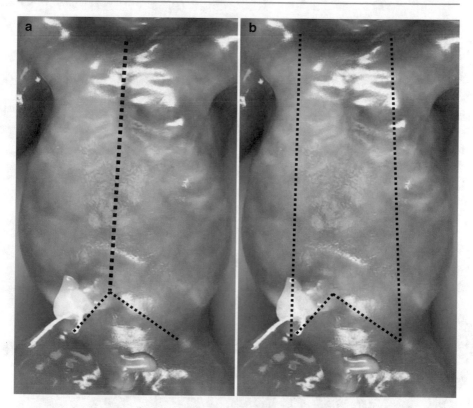

Fig. 6 Dissection types: classic, inverted Y cut (**a**), and inverted M type in first-trimester fetuses (**b**)

In malformed hearts, in addition to the diameter of the great vessels and their efferent vessels, various other measurements along the dissection are highly recommended:

– Tricuspid/mitral valve biometry
– Distance between tricuspid/mitral valve and apex
– Free wall thicknesses of left/right ventricles

If, for any reason, opening of the heart is postponed, the heart-lung block may be pre-fixed, allowing a possibility of a careful examination of pulmonary vessels, in particular, pulmonary venous return.

Lungs are examined in situ for segmentation and weighed. Samples may be taken for frozen tissue banking.

All abdominal viscera are primarily checked for situs prior to any dissection. After liver, spleen and pancreas examination are completed, the intestines are removed progressively by cutting the mesentery from the duodenum down.

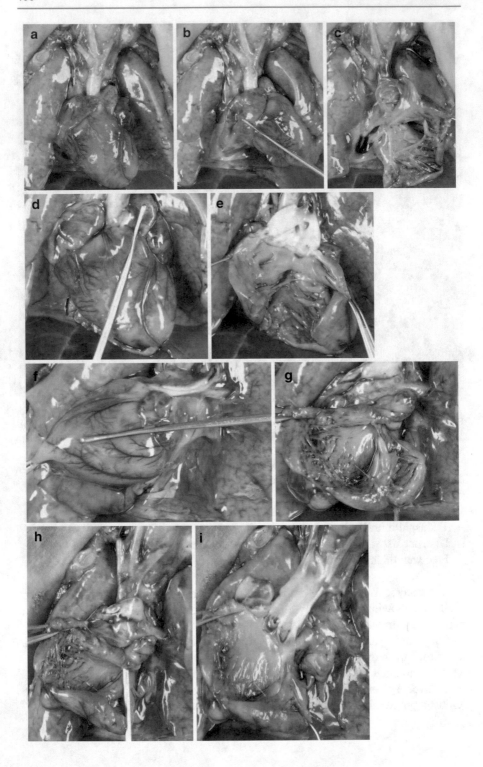

Fig. 7 Fetal heart dissection: Various views during fetal heart examination. View in situ (**a**) confirming normal ("N") position of great vessels, and their symmetrical diameters. (**b**) Moderately rotated to the left, this heart view shows systemic venous return, and the right atrium. (**c**) Right heart opening along the line depicted by the probe (**b**). Right auricle, tricuspid valve, and right ventricle are exposed. (**d**) The probe is dressed to show the next-step dissection to right ventricular outflow. (**e**) Right ventricular outflow with pulmonary infundibulum, and pulmonary trunk with two ostia for pulmonary artery branches. (**f**) The probe outlines the left ventricle cut lane from the pulmonary veins (left ones visible), through left auricle, mitral valve to the left ventricle. (**g**) Left ventricle view. (**h**) Probe is inserted in ascending aorta showing the next-step cut. (**i**) Left ventricular outflow showing mitro-aortic continuity and aortic valves with coronary ostia

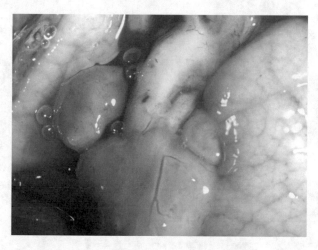

Fig. 8 First-trimester heart: 11-week heart in situ showing malposition ("D") of great vessels, and asymmetry with hypoplastic pulmonary artery

Before removing kidneys and adrenals, peritoneal dissection is necessary in order to allow better observation of renal vasculature and any other underlying anomaly. In autopsies limited to kidneys, in the context of anhydramnios, lumbar incisions allow extraction of the kidneys, and histology with biopsies for DNA studies (Fig. 9). One example of an oriented approach in fetal pathology represents small kidneys. If the renal hypoplasia with or without cystic renal disease is observed grossly, eyes should be dissected, to look for signs of retinal coloboma, identifying the *PAX2* gene in renal coloboma syndrome. Eye dissection, when indicated, is performed by sphenoidal windows from the cranial base.

The uterus and ovaries should be evaluated externally and included for histologic study. Testes after 30 weeks are examined from the inguinal canals, which are at first dilated with blunt scissors prior to removal with forceps.

If any anomaly is present, the thyroid gland should be dissected and included for histology preferentially by the transverse laryngeal cut at the same level. Esophagus and trachea are separated dorsally downward and a probe is inserted to assess esophageal permeability.

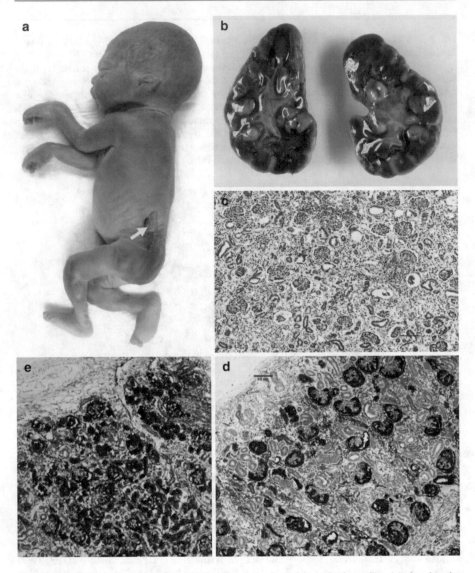

Fig. 9 Kidney-limited autopsy in a 25-week fetus terminated for anhydramnios: (**a**) showing the sole incision line (light blue arrow). (**b**) Moderately enlarged kidneys on gross/sagittal section. (**c**) HES (×20) histologic "glomerular crowding" in the cortex. (**d**) CD10 (×20) An absence of proximal tubules is evident compared to control (**e**), signing the diagnosis of tubular dysgenesis (homozygous *ACE* variants identified later)

Part 6: Neuropathology (Triage and Samplings)

Neuropathologic evaluations should be performed in the following cases:

– TOPs with any brain malformation seen on prenatal ultrasound scans
– TOPs without prenatal brain malformation, but in the context of syndromes without evident diagnosis

- IUFDs in the context of isolated or complex brain anomaly (expectative prenatal approach or parental TOP refusal)
- Term IUFDs

Pre-fixation in situ is performed systematically by injecting the zinc-formalin (4% formaldehyde) through anterior and posterior fontanels the day before autopsy. It allows better preservation and easier extraction even in cases of severe hydrocephalus. This procedure and other pre-analytic procedures may be performed by the technical staff.

To preserve head appearance as much as possible, the scalp incision is made dorsally from one ear to another. The postero-lateral downward cuts from each end of the previous incisions to the base of the neck allow better assessment of the brainstem and cerebellum. The skin flaps are then reflected frontally and posteriorly to expose cranial bones. Holding the fetal neck with the left hand, with fetal face forward, two incisions are first made on lateral sides of anterior fontanelle, and blunt scissors are carefully introduced, tangentially to the bone plan. The fetal head is rotated 180° and parasagittal incisions are made posteriorly on each side to maintain the falx cerebri. They are continued laterally to the parieto-occipital juncture. At this point blunt scissors are introduced in posterior fossa to cut the cerebellar falx. The fetal head is turned again 180° so that the operator faces the fetal back, and parasagittal incisions are prolonged frontally and fronto-parietally. Sectioning through frontal bone creates bone windows which might easily be removed. At that stage, the fetal head is reflected mildly to the back with a recipient dish held posteriorly. From the olfactory bulbs on, the cranial nerves are resected at the skull base, and the brain is progressively removed from the fetal skull.

If required, the spinal cord is preferentially removed by an anterior approach. In the lumbar region, the vertebral pedicles are divided with scalpel. Blunt scissors are introduced to the medullary canal and its opening upwards on each side exposes the spinal cord. Its removal is from the filum terminale by dissection of posterior nerve roots.

The brain and the spinal cord are fixed in microzinc-zinc formalin solution (formaldehyde 4%). Generally, extended fixation is necessary before a neuropathologic evaluation is performed (see Part III).

Part 7: Banking

For years it was stated that paraffin blocks are sufficient for DNA studies, until it became clear that formalin degrades DNA, reducing quality for most current NGS techniques.

It is consequently of the highest importance to systematically conserve frozen tissue for any ancillary molecular tests. In regard to resistance of autolysis, it is preferable to conserve lymphocyte-rich tissues such as thymus and spleen for DNA studies. Furthermore, fresh tissue biopsies (liver, lung, skin) are also used for various biochemical screens such as for sterol, lysosomal disorders, etc.

In cases of any suspicion of infectious fetopathy, polymerase chain reaction (PCR) probes (simplex or multiplex) may be ordered on frozen fetal tissue.

Part 8: Histology

Unlike gross-fetal organ examination, which closely resembles the postnatal state, varying predominantly by organ size, fetal histology is highly gestational age-dependent with major differences in histogenesis and histology from embryo to birth.

Very specific histological changes appear with each step of development, allowing the determination of developmental stage by studying fetal lungs, kidneys, and skin.

Briefly, fetal lung maturation is divided into four principal stages: (1) pseudoglandular (approx. 9–16 weeks), (2) canalicular (17–26 weeks), (3) saccular (27–32 weeks), and (4) alveolar (after 32 weeks) [16]. From the pseudoglandular stage onwards, successive subdivisions of airway structures occur, resulting in a complete conducting airway system during early childhood. Radial alveolar count (CRA) based on the terminal respiratory unit, i.e., air spaces distal to a terminal respiratory bronchiole, varies from 2.2 at 24–27 weeks to 4.4 at 40 weeks [17]. Although generally used to evaluate lung maturation in diaphragmatic hernia, other causes of lung hypoplasia, or failure to thrive, CRA may also provide information regarding developmental stage.

Even in macerated fetuses, assessment of age by nephrogenesis remains feasible by cortical glomerular generations' ray count on sagittal renal section, i.e., medullary ray glomerular counting [18]. At the age of 23 weeks, three layers of mature glomeruli in the cortical area are formed. Their number increases progressively by approximately one layer each additional week (Fig. 10).

Additionally, in skin biopsies at the age of 10 weeks no appendages are observed. At about 14 weeks budding of the basal cells appears. Sebaceous glands and hair shafts become visible at 16 weeks. Elongation of eccrine ducts is apparent at 23/24 weeks. Its coiling is seen only after 30 weeks [19].

The retention period in macerated IUFDs is estimated by an extension of the "loss of nuclear basophilia" (LONB) in various organs [20, 21, 22] (Table 1).

On a systematic basis, the following viscera are traditionally examined: lungs, thymus, liver, spleen, pancreas, kidneys, adrenals, and gonads. In fresh stillbirths (<48 h), heart histology (apex) is useful for evaluation of loss of nuclear basophilia (LONB).

Muscle histology is evaluated from several skeletal muscles, i.e., quadriceps/biceps/trapezius. It is important to take transverse sections to better evaluate fiber size, and to avoid false-positive results.

When indicated, bone histology is most often performed on the epiphyseal growth zone of the long bones, usually femoral or humeral, after decalcification. It is important to closely monitor decalcification procedure, which takes longer in older fetuses, in order to determine the optimal bone softness (for example via a needle test) for longitudinal cutting and embedding. In addition to classical H&E, Alcian Blue staining is frequently used.

Bone sutures or ribs may be sampled when indicated.

Fetal histogenesis is exhaustively described in a number of textbooks [23].

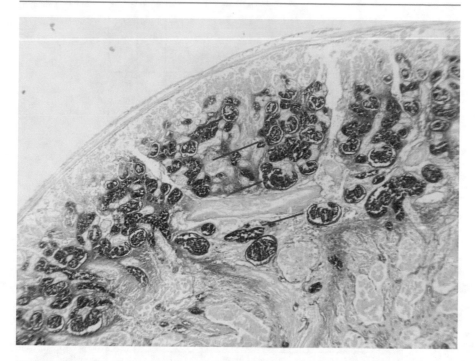

Fig. 10 Glomerular count. Fetal kidney at 24 weeks (CD10, ×20) showing high level of macera-tion with a diffuse loss of nuclear basophilia. However, number of mature glomeruli layers, labeled herein by CD10, is easily counted to 4

Part 9: Autopsy Report

One should always bear in mind that the autopsy report belongs to the family and will be read by them. It should be concise and written in clear language avoiding unnecessary jargon or terms. Terminology may be provided by the major online databases, allowing international standardization of autopsy reports.

Correlated by the above guidelines, only major or significant pathologic findings should be reported.

If, however, there are prenatally suspected diverse anomalies, absent on fetal pathology exam, they should be described as negative findings to clarify the clini-cians' dilemma.

Concerning the timing of postmortem reports, an initial, provisional report might be issued shortly following the autopsy if major macroscopic abnormalities are documented. In isolated congenital heart malformations (CHM), congenital dia-phragmatic hernia (CDH), or the most frequent chondrodysplasias, the X-rays or gross examination findings may be sufficient for the essential elements of the diag-nosis. These reports should be provided to the parents as soon as possible. In other cases, the results of all ancillary investigations should be incorporated into an over-all final postmortem examination report, with interpretation and comments.

Table 1 Determining the retention period from demise by studying loss of nuclear basophilia (LONB) in various fetal cells / organs

	≥4 h	≥8 h	≥18 h	≥24 h	≥36 h	≥48 h	≥72 h	≥96 h	≥1 week	≥2 week	≥4 week	≥8 week
Kidney	Cortical tubules LONB					Glomerular LONB					Complete LONB	
Lung			Bronchial epithelial detachment	Bronchial cartilage matrix LONB				Bronchial epithelial LONB	Tracheal cartilage LONB	Alveolar wall LONB		Complete LONB
Liver				Individual hepatocyte LONB				Complete LONB				
Heart				Inner half of myocardium LONB		Outer half of myocardium LONB						
G.I. tract		Mucosal epithelial LONB					Transmural LONB		Complete LONB			
Adrenal				Fetal adrenal cortex LONB			Adult adrenal cortex LONB		Complete LONB			
Pancreas					Complete LONB							

References

1. Eurin D. Atlas radiographique du squelette foetal normal. Paris: Lavoisier MSP; 1993.
2. Hall CM, Offiah AC, Forzano F, Lituania M, Fink M, Krakow D. Fetal and perinatal skeletal dysplasias: an atlas of multimodality imaging. 1st ed. London: CRC Press Radcliffe Publishing; 2012.
3. Dawood Y, Strijkers GJ, Limpens J, Oostra RJ. Novel imagingtechniques to study postmortem human fetal anatomy: a systematic review on microfocus-CT and ultra-high-field MRI. Eur Radiol. 2019;13:1–13.
4. Freimer N, Sabatti C. The human phenome project. Nat Genet. 2003;34(1):15–21.
5. Robinson PN, Kôhler S, Bauer S, Seelow D, Horn D, Mundlos S. The human phenotype ontology: a tool for annotating and analyzing human hereditary disease. Am J Hum Genet. 2008;83(5):610–5.
6. Robinson PN. Deep phenotyping for precise medicine. Hum Mutat. 2012;33:776–80.
7. Genest DR, Singer DB. Estimating the time of death in stillborn fetuses: III. External fetal examination; a study of 86 stillborns. Obstet Gynecol. 1992;80(4):593–600.
8. Pauli RM, Reiser CA, Lebovitz RM, Kirkpatrick SJ. Wisconsin Stillbirth Service Program: I. Establishment and assessment of a community-based program for etiologic investigation of intrauterine deaths. Am J Med Genet. 1994;50(2):116–34.
9. Pauli RM, Reiser CA. Wisconsin Stillbirth Service Program: II. Analysis of diagnoses and diagnostic categories in the first 1,000 referrals. Am J Med Genet. 1994;50(2):135–53.
10. Hansmann M. Ultrasonic diagnosis in obstetrics and gynecology. Berlin: Springer; 1985.
11. Merlob P, Sivan Y, Reisner SH. Anthropometric measurements of the newborn infant 27 to 41 gestational weeks. Birth Defects. 1984;20:7.
12. Mehes K. Inner canthal and intermammary indices in the newborn infant. J Pediatr. 1974;85:90.
13. Gripp KW, Slavotinek AM, Hall JG, Allanson JE. Handbook of physical measurements. Oxford: Oxford University Press; 2013.
14. Anderson RH, Becker AE, Freedom RM, et al. Sequential segmental analysis of congenital heart disease. Pediatr Cardiol. 1984;5:281–7.
15. Anderson RH, Becker AE. The heart: structure in health and disease. London: Gower Medical Publication; 1992.
16. Langston C, Kida K, Reed M, Thurlbeck WM. Human lung growth in late gestation and in the neonate. Am Rev Respir Dis. 1984;129:607.
17. Emery JL, Mithal A. The number of alveoli in the terminal respiratory unit of man during late intrauterine life and childhood. Arch Dis Child. 1960;35:544–7.
18. Hinchliffe SA, Sargent PH, Chan YF, van Velzen D, Howard CV, Hutton JL, Rushton DI. "Medullary ray glomerular counting" as a method of assessment of human nephrogenesis. Pathol Res Pract. 1992;188(6):775–82.
19. Ersch J, Stallmach T. Assessing gestational age from histology of fetal skin: an autopsy study of 379 fetuses. Obstet Gynecol. 1999;94(5 Pt 1):753–7.
20. Genest DR. Estimating the time of death in stillborn fetuses: II. Histologic evaluation of the placenta; a study of 71 stillborns. Obstet Gynecol. 1992;80(4):585–92.
21. Genest DR, Williams MA, Greene MF. Estimating the time of death in stillborn fetuses: I Histologic evaluation of fetal organs; an autopsy study of 150 stillborns. Obstet Gynecol. 1992;80(4):575–84.
22. Jacques SM, Qureshi F, Johnson A, Alkatib AA, Kmak DC. Estimation of time of fetal death in the second trimester by placental histopathological examination. Pediatr Dev Pathol. 2003;6(3):226–32.
23. Martinovic J. Urinary system: development and diseases. In: Khong TY, Malcomson RDG, editors. Keeling's fetal and neonatal pathology. Berlin: Springer; 2015.

Molecular Workup Guided by Fetal Examination

Jelena Martinovic and Neil J. Sebire

Part 10: Genetic Studies

Over the last few decades, genetics has made revolutionary advances in all medical fields, profoundly modifying the concept of diagnosis which has become molecular in a growing number of entities.

In the field of fetal pathology, an increasing number of developmental genes has been identified, as well as "adult" ones acting in their most severe forms from the embryo-fetal period.

Therefore, directing post-fetal pathology molecular studies by the multidisciplinary team has become an essential task for every developmental pathologist.

In many instances, such as in most common chondrodysplasias, fetal renal cystic diseases, etc., the molecular diagnosis is already suspected (on fetal radiograms, renal histology etc.), and targeted evaluation might be sufficient to allow genetic diagnosis and counseling. However, in many others, although fetal pathology might reveal additional data, not seen on prenatal scans, wider pan-genomic screening may be necessary to maximize the chance of obtaining a diagnosis.

It should be clear that with the expansion of genomic techniques, in a growing number of cases, aCGH or WES identifies de novo or inherited new variants, of unknown or uncertain predicted effect on phenotype. Without functional studies, it may frequently be impossible to determine clinical significance in the postmortem setting and diagnosis may be based on the fetal phenotype. Only rigorous analysis of both molecular data and the fetal phenotype, as well as saving tissue cultures for

J. Martinovic (✉)
Unit of Embryo-Fetal Pathology, University Hospitals AP-HP, Antoine Béclère,
Paris Saclay University, Clamart, France
e-mail: jelena.martinovic@aphp.fr

N. J. Sebire
Department of Histopathology, Great Ormond Street Hospital and ICH UCL, London, UK
e-mail: neil.sebire@gosh.nhs.uk

© Springer Nature Switzerland AG 2021
J. Martinovic (ed.), *Practical Manual of Fetal Pathology*,
https://doi.org/10.1007/978-3-030-42492-3_9

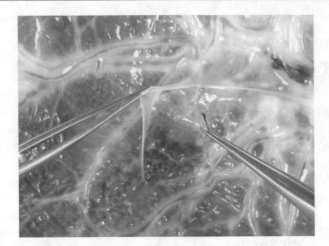

Fig. 1 Chorionic biopsy for postmortem karyotyping: close view of chorionic biopsy procedure including a detachment of an amniotic layer from the fetal surface away from chorionic vessels, and sampling of about 5–10 mm in diameter of chorion. While pulling up the chorion, chorionic villi should be separated from chorion from underneath by scissors

functional studies, allows definite incrimination of such variants as causal and hence allows appropriate prenatal diagnosis in future pregnancies.

It is noteworthy that the establishment of fetal karyotype and/or array CGH is almost always currently first-line test prior to requesting further genomic study. If not performed during the prenatal period, karyotype can be established on the chorionic biopsy of the fresh placenta (Fig. 1) or on any fetal tissue (lungs, skin, etc.). aCGH might be solicited simultaneously or subsequently on the frozen tissue biopsies.

Part 11: Post-fetal Autopsy Counseling

A genetic counselor, belonging to the lab staff or to a multidisciplinary fetal medical unit, is of benefit since there are growing numbers of available molecular diagnoses requiring understanding and discussion of adequate pre- and post-analytic information that the parents should be offered. Moreover, in most of genomic tests, the trio consisting of the fetal and parental DNAs is recommended and improves diagnostic yield.

General Considerations

Cost-efficiency of each fetopathology unit is monitored closely by the department of finances. For practical purposes, it has been established in France that 100 fetal autopsies/year at a third level care maternity, i.e., mostly TOPs, should be handled by one full-time faculty member.

Thus, it is important to individually design the best model for each department's efficiency. The delegation of certain parts of the protocol to a dedicated and well-trained technical staff is an option. Obviously, the technical staff should be covered under the medical liability.

Summary

In summary, every effort should be made to enhance access to the full range of modern methods of fetopathologic examination and investigation after death in pre-defined indications. Despite the considerable progress in prenatal imaging and pregnancy surveys in the last decades, there remains value in pathologic and molecular analysis to ensure adequate genetic counseling, including patients who have been admitted to intensive care units (ICUs) [1]. In a meta-analysis of 31 reported clinico-pathologic studies, around 30% diagnostic discordancy has been reported [2] similar to unpublished data from a 5-year audit of fetuses from one of the author's tertiary-level care maternity unit (JM, unpublished data).

Despite this evidence, many centers continue to face difficulties in either service provision or uptake rates. Close cross talks with clinicians and constant efforts in clinico-pathologic continuing education are necessary to provide an optimal environment for the development of fetal pathology.

Bibliography

1. Combes A, Mokhtari M, Couvelard A, et al. Clinical and autopsy diagnosis in the intensive care unit. Arch Intern Med. 2004;164(4):389–92.
2. Winters B, Custer J, Galvagno SM, et al. Diagnostic errors in the intensive care unit: a systematic review of autopsy studies. BMJ Qual Saf. 2012;21(11):894–902.

Part IV

Neurofetopathological Examination

Abstract

Brain malformations are deviations in anatomy and/or histology occurring during embryofetal development. Like an aircraft's "black box," the malformed brain records critical information on the *ubi quando quomodo* of what went wrong during the development of the central nervous system (CNS). These questions are at the center of the problematic of neurodevelopmental disorders. They are amenable to analysis through a neuropathological examination. This examination should be mandatory in fetal losses, either spontaneous or after pregnancy termination. But it should be performed in accordance with strict current legal and ethical rules. Finally neurofetopathological examination requires very good knowledge of the "origami" of neurodevelopment process and its underlying molecular signalling pathways.

Abbreviations

CNS	Central nervous system
CP	Cortical plate
CRC	Cajal–Retzius cell
CST	Cortico-spinal tract
CV	Cresyl-violet
GE	Ganglionic eminence
H&E	Hematoxylin & Eosin
IPC	Inner progenitor cell
IZ	Intermediate zone
OPC	Outer progenitor cell
PC	Postconceptual age
RG	Radial glia

RGC   Radial glia cells
SVZ   Subventricular zone
VZ   Ventricular zone
WD   Weeks of development
WG   Weeks gestation

Methodology

Ferechte Encha-Razavi

Abbreviations

CNS	Central nervous system
CP	Cortical plate
CRC	Cajal–Retzius cell
CST	Cortico-spinal tract
CV	Cresyl-Violet
GE	Ganglionic eminence
H&E	Hematoxylin & eosin
IPC	Inner progenitor cell
IZ	Intermediate zone
OPC	Outer progenitor cell
PC	Postconceptual age
RG	Radial glia
RGC	Radial glia cells
SVZ	Subventricular zone
VZ	Ventricular zone
WD	Weeks of development
WG	Weeks gestation

A successful neuropathological examination depends first of all on a good preservation of the cerebral tissue. The usual problem in fetal pathology is the rapid brain autolysis due to retention in utero, either after spontaneous death or pregnancy termination, as well as to the delay between delivery and CNS extraction. In situ

F. Encha-Razavi (✉)
Unité d'Embryofoetopathologie, Hôpital Universitaire Necker-Enfants malades, Paris, France
e-mail: ferechte.razavi@aphp.fr

© Springer Nature Switzerland AG 2021
J. Martinovic (ed.), *Practical Manual of Fetal Pathology*,
https://doi.org/10.1007/978-3-030-42492-3_10

fixation may help tissue conservation in case of a delivery outside opening hours (see Chapter Martinovic, Sebire). A good knowledge of the pregnancy follow-up (fetal imaging, biological, genetic and cytogenetic analysis …), as well as the parents' medical past history and family tree is required to orient brain examination and the extent of samplings.

CNS Extraction

Before CNS extraction, defects of the scalp, skull, face, and eyes should be described and photographed. Tissue samples from frontal and/or occipital poles and salient pathological regions (tumor, aneurysm, dysplasia) are frozen at −80° for further molecular study.

Brain

In fetuses, brain extraction is performed according to a common method developed for newborns (see "Consent for Medical Autopsy" chapter). However, because the extreme fragility of fetal brain due to lack of myelin and to a very high concentration of water (70%) a special "tour de main" is useful for tissue preservation. To protect the brain, our practice is to perform CNS extraction in a recipient filled with clear water. After excision of the scalp and the sutures, the brain is examined in situ to search for external hydrocephalus and brain atrophy. Then the cranial vault is closed using the scalp as a "bag," while the body is turned upside down in the recipient. A gentle traction on the brain allows a better visualization of the basal structures (cranial nerves, pituitary stalk, and the hexagon of Willis). In addition, it allows resecting the brain stem as far as possible beyond its boundary with the cervical spinal cord. Samples from the upper spinal cord are informative to study lower cortico-spinal tracts and pyramids decussation. Once in the water, the brain may be manipulated easily to search for external defects. Importantly, water immersion by filling superficial cavities and cystic pouches allows to visualize arachnoidal cysts and the parenchymal lamination (hydranencephaly, porencephaly). Then, the brain is transferred to a large container for fixation being attached through the basilar artery. The basal cranium is analyzed further to search for ethmoidal defects (lack of crista galli apophysis, anterior neural tube defects, tumoral mass), as well as defects of the sella turcica (hypophyseal and hypothalamic tumors) and hypoplasia/aplasia of semi-circular canals.

Spinal Cord

Extraction of the spinal cord is compulsory in the context of CNS malformations and primary fetal akinesia. This could be performed by dorsal laminectomy by cutting through the pedicles and lifting the vertebral arches from the vertebral bodies therefore exposing the dura matter. The spinal cord is entirely removed and transferred into a fixative container and processed until the paraffin stage. Cross sections are cut later on during paraffin embedding.

For a better identification of the spinal cord levels, we prefer to remove the entire spinal cord, using a ventral approach. The piece is then decalcified and cut through the intervertebral disks leaving the cord intact. In addition, it gives a good indication on the level of the spinal cord. In particular, it allows viewing the entire spinal canal and the dural sac (useful in case of myelomeningocele).

Eyes

As part of the CNS, eyes must always be examined in case of brain malformations. They have to be removed, fixed in formalin zinc, then measured, cut and sampled. We usually practice antero-posterior para-sagittal sections. This allows to perform a global examination of the eyes as well as of the optic nerves.

Fixation

Concerning fixation of the CNS, different practices do exist. We use 2–4 weeks' immersion into commercial formalin zinc 4% solution (Microzinc). When a parental consent for research is obtained, paraformaldehyde (PFA) and/or −80° conservation may be used.

Photographs

Photographic documentation is crucial for a proper prospective (as well as retrospective) neuropathological interpretation. They should be captured on a perfectly clean, transparent board (plexiglass or glass) settled above a blue (or light green) hard sheet with metric reference (Fig. 1). The entire process of neuropathological examination must be captured, before, during, and after extraction as well as after fixation of the brain. Before removal of the brain, external defects such as facial clefts, scalp aplasia, bulging masse, and anomalies of the calvarium (suture distention or fusion…) are photographed. During brain extraction, cystic formation, a discrepancy between a large cranium and a small brain (external hydrocephalus), and any salient pathological feature should be captured in situ. We take pictures from the basal cranium after removal of the brain. During macroscopical examination, pictures of the external shape and the internal configuration of the fixed cerebral hemispheres are required, namely dorsal, lateral, and basal views as well as the ventral and dorsal views of the brain stem and the cerebellum. Microscopical slides may be scanned entirely or salient pathological features can be captured using a photomicroscope.

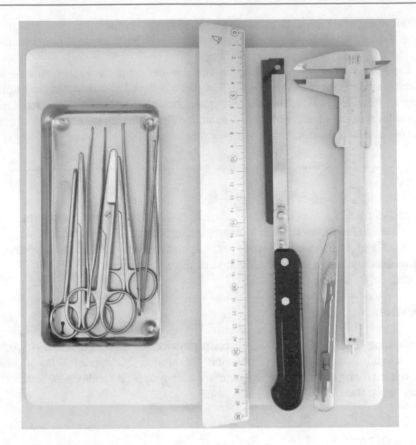

Fig. 1 Material for macroscopical examination of the central nervous system

Macroscopical Examination

After 2–4 weeks fixation, macroscopical examination followed by tissue sampling for histological analysis is performed. The examination of the formalin fixed brain is performed after a whole night rincage in clear water. Four steps are required: photographic pictures, biometric evaluation, cutting, and sampling.

Biometry

Measurements are the most reliable criteria for an evaluation of the brain maturation. The brain is weighed without the falx cerebri. The fronto-occipital length of each hemisphere and the transversal distance of the cerebellum are recorded. Evaluation is made in relation to the body weight and gestational age, using special charts adapted to fetuses (see **"Fetal Biometry"** of Hargitai). The transverse distance of cerebellar hemispheres increases 1 mm a week until 20th WG and grows faster beyond this stage.

External Shape

The gyral pattern is examined on the lateral wall of cerebral hemispheres. At the basal surface of the brain, the cranial nerves, the pituitary stalk, and the afferent vessels of the brain (Willis circle) are checked. The region of the pituitary stalk is carefully examined in search of a hypothalamic hamartoma (Fig. 2).

Internal Configuration

Examination of the internal configuration of the brain requires brain cutting. We start brain cutting with the resection of the brain stem and the cerebellum at the level of the midbrain, between the superior and inferior colliculi (Fig. 3). An additional rostral slice including the superior colliculi is made. Then, the cerebral hemispheres are cut. In fetuses above 20th WG, we perform first a sagittal section (Fig. 4). This allows examining the midline structures mainly the size and the morphology of the corpus callosum. Measurements of the length and width of the corpus callosum are performed at the level of rostrum, corpus, and splenium. Then, coronal sections (frontal) are performed, namely at the level of the frontal lobes, mammillary bodies, mid-pons (Charcot level), pulvinar and occipital lobes (Fig. 5).

Tissue Sampling for Histological Study

Small sections are adequate before <20th WG. Later, whole mount histological sections allow a better topographical examination. The minimal number of sections we recommend in macroscopically normal brain are from the mammillary bodies or from the mid-pons levels including the fronto-parietal, the thalamus-hippocampus, and the basal ganglia. From the brain stem, we recommend sections between the colliculi and the mid medulla oblongata (Figs. 6, 7, and 8). The pons is examined with the cerebellum, one half sagittally and the other half transversally. The spinal cord is examined at the cervical, low thoracic, and lumbar levels. Additional blocks are taken from the areas where salient pathological changes exist. Small sections are cut at 7 μm and large ones at 10 μm. In case of brain autolysis, despite apparent liquefaction sampling could be performed. Brain tissue is surprisingly well preserved.

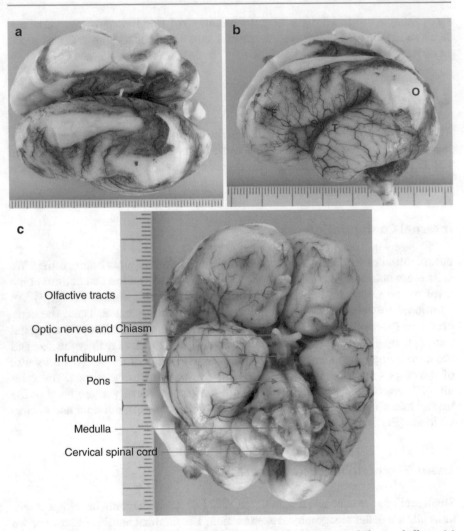

Olfactive tracts

Optic nerves and Chiasm

Infundibulum

Pons

Medulla

Cervical spinal cord

Fig. 2 External appearance of the cerebral hemispheres, brain stem, and the cerebellum: (**a**) Dorsal view of the cerebral hemispheres separated by the deep dorsal interhemispheric sulcus, (**b**) Lateral view of the left cerebral hemisphere. *F* frontal lobe, *P* parietal lobe, *T* temporal lobe, *O occipital lobe*, *SV* Sylvian valley, (**c**) Basal view of rhe cerebral hemispheres

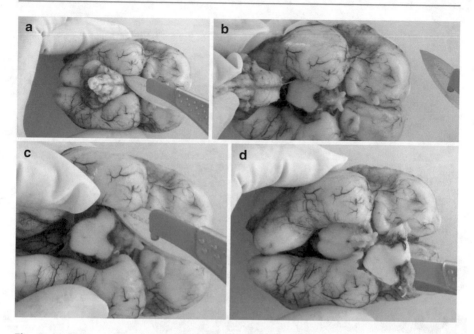

Fig. 3 (**a, b**) Resection of the brain stem in between the colliculi; (**c, d**) sampling of the mesencephalon

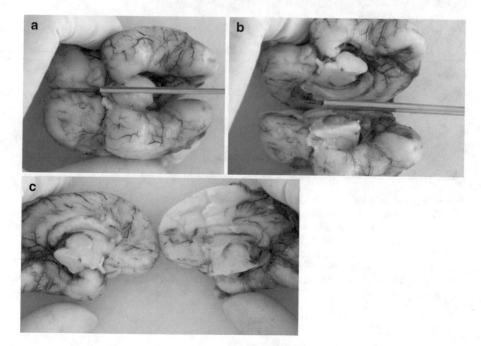

Fig. 4 (**a, b**) Medial sagittal section of the cerebral hemispheres; (**c**) antero-posterior view of the midline structures including the three segments of the corpus callosum (rostrum, corpus, splenium) and the septum pilars

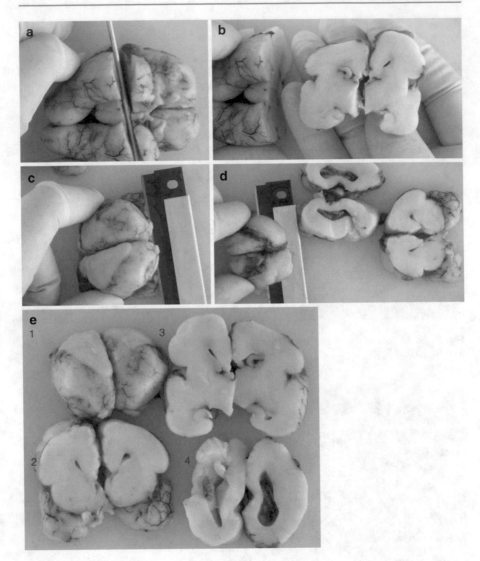

Fig. 5 Antero-posterior coronal sections of the cerebral hemispheres: (**a**) first section at the level of mid-pons; (**b**) Examination of the two halves of cerebral hemispheres; (**c, d**) Additional sections of the anterior and posterior halves; (**e**) Composite figure of coronal anterior to posterior sections of cerebral hemispheres showing (1) the frontal poles with olfactory tracts; (2) the frontal lobes with the lateral ventricles and the rostrum of the corpus callosum; (3) cerebral hemispheres at the level of mammillary bodies showing the ventricular system, the midline structure (corpus callosum and cavum), the ganglionic eminence, the basal ganglia, the sylvian T-shape fissure, hippocampus; (4) the occipital horns

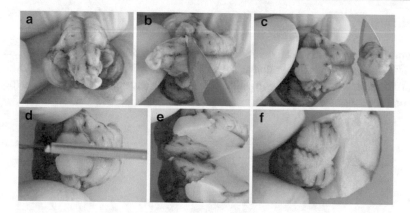

Fig. 6 Brain stem and cerebellum examination: (**a**) ventral view of the brain stem and the cerebellar hemispheres showing the vertebral and basilar arteries, the pontic relief, the medulla, and cervical spinal cord, (**b**) section of the medulla (**c**) indentification of the pyramidal tracts and the inferior olives (**d–f**) sagittal sections of the brain stem and the vermis

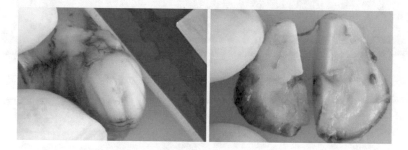

Fig. 7 Axial sections of the brain stem and cerebellum

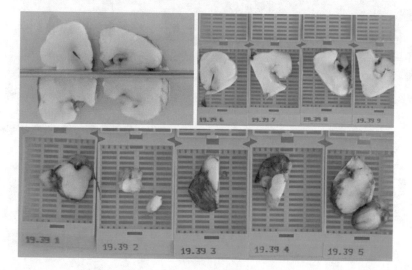

Fig. 8 Sampling of cerebral hemispheres, brain stem, and cerebellum

Staining

Hematoxylin & Eosin (H&E) stains are our preference for routine diagnosis. Cresyl-Violet (CV) is an excellent nuclear marker useful for the evaluation of migrational disorders and neurodegeneration. Immunohistochemical study is performed depending on the context.

How to Examine a Brain in Development

Ferechte Encha-Razavi

Fetal brain examination implies an acute knowledge of the timing and the development of the nervous system during gestation. The first half of gestation corresponds to the neurulation, differentiation of cerebral vesicles, and corticogenesis. The second half is characterized by the tremendous expansion of the cerebral cortex leading to the cerebral hemispheres' growth and the gyral formation.

Ventricular System

The ventricular system develops from the cavities of embryonic cerebral vesicles after closure of the neural tube. It undergoes a gradual narrowing. The cavity of the rhombencephalon, with its thin roof, forms the fourth ventricle. The aqueduct of Sylvius results from the narrowing of the mesencephalon cavity, while the diencephalon and telencephalon cavities form the third and lateral ventricles, respectively, communicating through the foramen of Monro. Until 18th WG hemispheres show a vesicular aspect with thin walls and large ventricles. As development proceeds, the ventricular system undergoes gradual narrowing and becomes slit-shaped at term. However, a physiological hydrocephalus of the occipital horns persists until the 24th WG and may be present in young premature babies (colpocephaly). In fetuses, the cavity between the two leaves of the septum pellucidum forms the *cavum septi pellucidi* and the *cavum vergae,* respectively. Its wall has no ependyma and consists of fibrillary elements and large macrophagic cells. The cavum shrinks at the end of pregnancy and disappears after birth.

F. Encha-Razavi (✉)
Unité d'Embryofoetopathologie, Hôpital Universitaire Necker-Enfants malades, Paris, France
e-mail: ferechte.razavi@aphp.fr

© Springer Nature Switzerland AG 2021
J. Martinovic (ed.), *Practical Manual of Fetal Pathology*,
https://doi.org/10.1007/978-3-030-42492-3_11

Choroïd Plexus

Choroid plexus formation follows a postero-anterior gradient. The first primordium of choroid plexus is formed at the 6th weeks post-conception (WPC) in the roof of the fourth ventricle, by a folding of the leptomeninges covered with the underlying neuroepithelium. Primordiums of the lateral ventricles and the third ventricle occur between the 7th and the 8th WPC, respectively. Based on the shape of the plexus and the appearance of the epithelium, four stages have been recognized. A pseudostratified neuroepithelium is described in the first stage (7th to 9th WPC). During Stage II (from the 10th WPC to the 16th WG), the plexus becomes lobulated. They reach their maximum size at about the 12th WG and fill the entire lateral ventricle and the choroidal epithelium becomes simple and low columnar. Toward the end of stage III (between the 17th and the 28th WG), the loose mesenchyme in the stroma is replaced by loose connective tissue containing cysts devoid of epithelial lining that may be visualized by ultrasonography. These cysts regress spontaneously in most cases between the 20th and the 24th WG. During stage IV (from the 29th WG until term), the lining epithelium becomes cuboidal with well-developed blood vessels and connective tissue.

Cerebral Wall

Except for the microglial cells, all the neuro-glial constituents of the CNS derive from the neuroepithelium, a pseudostratified layer of stem cells (also called radial glia cells), lining the neural tube. Neuroblasts formation relies at least on two waves of progenitor cells replication, occurring first in the ventricular zone, then in the subventricular zone and called the inner and outer progenitor cells (IPC, OPC), respectively. Mitosis occurs in the neuroepithelium with a characteristic inner-outer cycle (replication occurs in the apical zone under the arachnoid and division occurs in the basal zone in the ventricular region). By the 6th WPC, the hemispheric wall consists of a thick germinal subependymal layer or matrix, separated from the apical pia matter by a superficial acellular zone, called the marginal or molecular layer. By the 7th WPC, the outward migration of neuroblasts (cells with a neuronal fate) starts along the apical processes of the radial glia cells, called radial glia (RG). The RG processes extend from the ventricular zone to the basement membrane under the pia matter, where they constitute the superficial gliomesenchymal tissue, called glia limitans. The integrity of the radial glia scaffold made of vimentin positive parallel fibers is crucial for the upward displacement of migrating neurons (radial migration), produced by the continued cell proliferation of the germinal layer. By the 8th WPC, waves of migrating cells lead to the formation of a superficial highly cellular ribbon or cortical plate (CP), separated from the deep germinal layer by an intermediate zone (IZ), containing concentric waves and parallel rows of cells. In addition to migrating cells, the IZ contains the second generation of progenitor cells, called the outer progenitor cells (OPC). Between the 24th and the 40th WG, with the completion of the inside-out neuronal migration, the CP displays the horizontal and columnar stratifications characteristic of the human neocortex. The first wave of migrating neuroblasts forms the deepest cortical layer, while the latter constitutes the most superficial one. The IZ filled with projection fibers and tracts increases in width and forms the white matter at the same time. After completion of migration, islets of migrating cells may be found in the IZ (the periventricular white matter) and in the frontal lobe. Not to be mistaken for heterotopias.

Fetal Cortex

Fetal cortex displays two transient developmental features. (1) A superficial granular layer under the leptomeninges, the so-called Arnbrün layer, appearing between the 13th and the 14th WD and disappearing by the 27th to the 39th WG. However, remainings of the superficial granular layer may persist in term infants at the inferior border of the temporal and orbital cortex. (2) Cells of Cajal–Retzius (Cajal–Retzius cell, CRC), characteristic of the fetal cortex, appear in the molecular layer during embryonic period and disappear at term. They are considered as instrumental for the inside-out order of the cortical cellular organization.

"Status verrucosus" are tufts occurring in the cerebral cortex of fetuses below 24th WG. They are considered as artifacts due to brain fixation without meninges.

Ganglionic Eminence

In the dorsal telencephalon, neuronal migration takes place until depletion of the ventricular germinal layer. Simultaneously in the ventral telencephalon, tightly packed immature cells form voluminous germinal zones, called ganglionic eminences (GE). Depletion of the GE starts during the second half of gestation. They feed the fetal cortex in GABAergic interneurons and constitute the basal ganglia. They disappear at term.

Gyral Formation

The pattern of brain sulcation is a good marker of brain maturation and malformations (see Chap. 10, Fig 2). At the level of cerebral hemispheres, interhemispheric dorsal and ventral sulci may be identified as soon as 10th WG. Their presence rules out the diagnosis of classical form of holoprosencephaly. The establishment of the primary sulci follows an invariable schedule. The brain is smooth until the 18th WG. Primary fissures appear between the 18th and the 28th WG. Among them, Rolando (or central) and calcarine fissures occur first around 18th WG, followed by the parieto-occipital fissure. Operculization of the sylvian fossa begins at the 18th WG. By the 24th to the 28th WG, the superior temporal sulci (or T1) are established. Secondary sulci appear between the 28th and the 37th WG; they are quite variable.

How to Examine a Brain in Maldevelopment

Ferechte Encha-Razavi

Brain malformations are congenital deviations in anatomy and/or histology. They are related to a failure of the neurodevelopmental process with a primary event resulting in a pleiotropic cascade of secondary anomalies. A significant number of brain anomalies are malformative due to chromosomal and genetic abnormalities. Genetic factors interfere with the neurodevelopmental processes by disregulating specific signalling pathways. On the other hand, signalling pathways may be possible targets for exogenous disruptive factors, mimicking therefore similar pattern of malformations (phenocopy). By definition, secondary malformations cannot be inherited. However, inherited factors can predispose to secondary malformations.

The Checkup Procedure

To go further into the identification of neurodevelopmental disorders, a five-step checkup is necessary.

First, Describe

A detailed macroscopical and histological description of brain anomalies should be performed in details and the report should be understandable by a "nonspecialist." The macroscopical report must include information about (1) the growth of the CNS, (2) the external shape of the cerebral hemispheres, the brainstem, and the cerebellum, and (3) the internal configuration of the brain.

F. Encha-Razavi (✉)
Unité d'Embryofoetopathologie, Hôpital Universitaire Necker-Enfants malades, Paris, France
e-mail: ferechte.razavi@aphp.fr

© Springer Nature Switzerland AG 2021
J. Martinovic (ed.), *Practical Manual of Fetal Pathology*,
https://doi.org/10.1007/978-3-030-42492-3_12

The histological examination should focus at the level of cerebral walls (also called dorsal telencephalon, neopallium), the ventricular and subventricular zones (VZ, SVZ), the intermediate zone (IZ), and the cortical plate (CP). Examination should also describe midline structures, mainly the corpus callosum crossing tracts, the cavum, and the septal apparatus. At the level of the diencephalon (also called ventral telencephalon) the ganglionic eminences are described, as well as the basal nuclei and the anterior and posterior arms of the internal capsule. At the mesencephalic level, the colliculi (superior and inferior), the roof (called tectum) as well as the subcommissural organ just above the aqueduct of Sylvius are examined. An evaluation of the cranial nerve's nuclei (the III the oculomotor nerve and the IV the trochlear) should follow. The longitudinal cortico-spinal tracts (CST) are followed from the mesencephalic level to the medulla oblongata, where they form pyramids. Sagittal sections of the pons and the cerebellum allow to appreciate the pontine relief as well as the vermian foliation and lamination. On transversal sections of the hemi-pons, growth of tegmentum is compared to the basilar pons and pontic nuclei and projections are examined. At the level of the medulla, the superior olivary nuclei and the nuclei of XII cranial nerves (hypoglossal) have to be analyzed particularly in case of fetal akinesia and mandibular hypoplasia. At the level of the cervical spinal cord, the global architecture and the organization of the longitudinal tracts as well as the pyramids decussation are examined. In addition, the cellularity and integrity of the motoneurons is assessed. In the cerebellar hemispheres, lamination and deep nuclei (dentate and fastigial) are analyzed.

Two, Focus on the Primary Event

Brain malformations correspond to an arrest at a particular stage of the developmental process resulting in a failure of the following developmental stages. For instance, corpus callosum defects may result from an abnormal crossing or from a deficit in callosal fibers formation. In the first case identification of bundles of aberrant fibers (called Probst Bundles) confirms the axonal guidance defect and in the second a cortical malformation may explain the lack or reduction of callosal fibers resulting in agenesis or dysgenesis.

Three, Identify a Pathogenic Mechanism

For example, in the context of hydrocephalus, neuropathological evaluation may assign the malformation to the obliteration of the arachnoid space due to a neuroglial overmigration. Gaps in the glia limitans result in overmigration. The gaps may result from a damage to the brain or due to a developmental basement membrane defect.

Four, Recognize a Syndrome

For instance in fetuses, hydrocephalus due to overmigration when associated to cerebellar or ocular dysplasia and a meningoencephalocele is strongly suggestive of the Walker–Warburg syndrome part of the COMD (cerebro-oculo-muscular dysplasia) community, characteristic of alpha-dystroglycanopathies.

Five, Orient Genetic Studies

Neuropathological study by pointing out to a precise gene or a genetic cascade or to a community of pathogenetic events allows to save time and cost. For example, it could be conclusive when molecular investigations of a specific gene or a panel of genes are performed. In addition, neuropathological findings may facilitate the interpretation of pathogenic variations found by NGS.

Conclusion

Neurofetopathological examination requires a very good knowledge of the "origami" of neurodevelopmental process and its underlying molecular signalling pathways. Normal brain formation results from a cascade of biological and mechanical events driven by genetic and epigenetic factors. Genetic mutations disrupt these signalling pathways, which are also possible targets of exogenous factors such as virus, alcohol, hyperglycemia, and teratogens, thus mimicking similar phenotype (e.g., holoprosencephaly, microcephaly). For further identification of congenital neurodevelopmental defects, a five-step procedure is proposed:

First, describe
Two, focus on the primary event
Three, identify the underlying mechanism
Four, recognize a syndrome
Five, orient genetic studies

Acknowledgements My special thanks to Professor Michel VEKEMANS for his critical reading of this chapter and suggestions.

Part V

Placenta

Abstract

Assessment of placental growth, architecture, and histopathology can play an important role in understanding fetal well-being at all stages of pregnancy. In selected cases, it can provide specific diagnoses with treatment implications for mother or infant, predict recurrence risks, and guide the management of future pregnancies. However, these benefits can only be realized if the appropriate placentas are submitted to pathology with a relevant clinical history, evaluated in a timely manner by experts trained in perinatal pathology, and reported in a format understood by all key members of the health care team.

This chapter will provide essentials for optimal placenta exam at different stages of pregnancy with an update on principal occurring pathologies.

Introduction and Early Fetal Stage Placenta (First Trimester, 8–12 Gestational Weeks (WG))

Raymond W. Redline and Sanjita Ravishankar

Introduction

Examination of the placenta is an important tool for understanding adverse pregnancy outcomes. Best practice suggests that placental tissues from all pregnancies ending either spontaneously or for medical indications before 37 weeks be submitted for pathologic evaluation. Indications for submission after 37 weeks range from liberal to conservative and are the focus of two recent policy statements [1, 2]. These guidelines ensure a detailed and accurate recording of pathologically confirmed pregnancies by gestational age, developmental stage, and pathophysiologic category which can be very useful for subsequent clinical management and genetic counseling. It also ensures that, based on the pathologic findings, appropriate follow-up testing of the mother, fetus, or placenta can be initiated.

Placentas and early pregnancy specimens are best examined promptly without fixation by pathologists with an interest and special training in perinatal pathology. While useful information can be obtained from specimens refrigerated for 7 days (or more), expedited processing and reporting increases the opportunity for diagnoses to immediately benefit the mother and/or infant. Submission to pathology after fixation in formalin is a less desirable option, since the range of possible ancillary diagnostic tests may be limited. It is also obviously important that pathologists be provided with an accurate and complete patient history including gestational age, previous obstetric history, important aspects of the current pregnancy, birthweight, Apgar scores, relevant findings in the delivered fetus/infant, and the specific questions that the clinical care team would like the pathologist to address.

R. W. Redline (✉) · S. Ravishankar
Perinatal, Pediatric, and Gynecologic Pathology, Case Western Reserve University School of Medicine, University Hospitals Cleveland Medical Center, Cleveland, OH, USA
e-mail: raymondw.redline@Uhhospitals.org

© Springer Nature Switzerland AG 2021
J. Martinovic (ed.), *Practical Manual of Fetal Pathology*,
https://doi.org/10.1007/978-3-030-42492-3_13

Placental pathology is far too vast field to be reviewed meaningfully in a single chapter, so we will focus on placental findings that can help explain fetal abnormalities and pregnancy losses at all stages of gestation. It has been estimated that cause of death can be attributed to a placental cause in up to 60% of stillbirths [3], but nuanced consideration of this figure is important. While placentas do sometimes have primary abnormalities that by themselves explain morbidity and mortality (high grade lesions), they more frequently show a set of less severe (low grade) lesions and reaction patterns that may interact with genetic and environmental factors. All placental findings, together with their time of onset and duration, should be integrated with clinical data to provide the most likely explanation for an adverse outcome in each specific case.

The format of this chapter will be to consider placental findings by stage of pregnancy, but it should be emphasized that these distinctions are somewhat artificial and that few histopathologic sequences are restricted to one stage of pregnancy alone. To reinforce this point, Table 1 estimates the relative frequency of each of the specific histopathologic sequences described in this chapter at each stage of pregnancy.

Early Fetal Stage Placenta (First Trimester, 8–12 Gestational Weeks (WG))

Adverse Outcomes/Clinical Presentations

Spontaneous miscarriage (abortion):
- Threatened: vaginal bleeding without passage of tissue
- Incomplete: vaginal bleeding and passage of tissue
- Complete: passage of the entire chorionic sac

Missed "abortion":
- Anembryonic pregnancy: no fetal pole by ultrasound or histopathology
- Nodular/stunted embryo: major alteration of body plan
- Early fetal death: anatomically normal or with anomalies

Gestational trophoblastic disease:
- Complete hydatidiform mole: diandric diploidy
- Partial hydatidiform mole: diandric triploidy
- Trophoblast hyperplasia, nonspecific: rare trisomies, others
  Recurrent miscarriage: two or more consecutive first trimester losses

Approach to the Gross Specimen

Placental tissue from the early fetal stage is usually recognizable as a single loosely cohesive, three-dimensional tissue fragment, pale and spongy, often with some filmy attached membranes. This fragment is often obscured and must be

Table 1 Estimated relative frequency by stage of pregnancy of specific important histopathologic sequences

Placental lesion	1st trimester	2nd trimester	Early 3rd trimester	Late 3rd trimester
Uniformly hydropic avascular villi	++	0	0	0
Diffuse intervillous hemorrhage	++	0	0	0
Dysmorphic villi c/w aneusomy	++	+	+	Rare
Chronic histiocytic intervillositis	++	+	+	+
Chronic marginal abruption (venous)	+	++	++	+
Placental hydrops (edema)	+	++	++	+
Chronic villitis, infectious (TORCH)	Rare	++	++	+
Premature amnion/membrane rupture	+	++	++	+
Massive subchorial thrombohematoma	Rare	+	+	Rare
Acute chorioamnionitis	0	+	++	+
Maternal vascular malperfusion	0	Rare	++	+
Diffuse perivillous fibrin(oid) (MFI)	+	+	++	+
Findings c/w genetic/metabolic disease	Rare	+	++	+
Monochorionic twin vascular abnormalities	Rare	+	++	+
Fetal vascular malperfusion	0	Rare	+	++
Chronic villitis, idiopathic (VUE)	Rare	Rare	Rare	++
Fetal-stromal vascular maldevelopment	0	Rare	+	++
Fetal hemorrhage (normoblastemia)	0	Rare	+	++
Meconium-associated myonecrosis	0	0	0	++

"fished out" from amongst the abundant flat sheets of pale, decidualized endometrium (shiny on one side and rough like a "shag rug" on the other), dark hemorrhagic/necrotic tissue, and blood clots that constitute the majority of the specimen. Visualization with a hand lens or dissecting microscope after removal of attached blood and floating the tissue in saline can accentuate the multi-order branching pattern typical of chorionic villi and be useful for ensuring that the tissue submitted for cytogenetic analysis contains fetal-derived tissues (Fig. 1a). Fragmented fetal tissue or, on occasion, an intact degenerating nodular or stunted embryo or umbilical cord may also be identified amongst the placental and endometrial fragments and is carefully examined both macroscopically and microscopically for abnormalities.

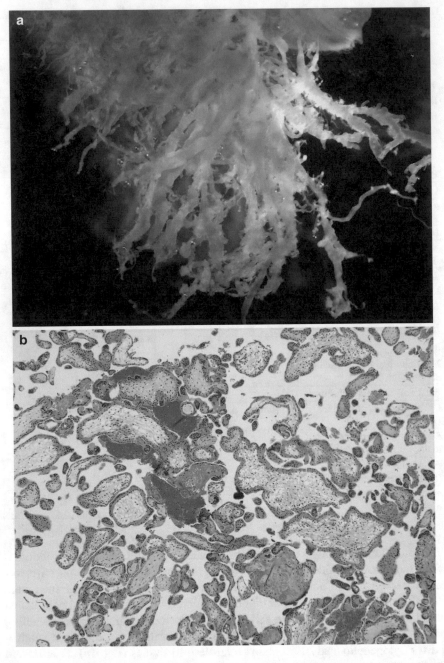

Fig. 1 First trimester placental pathology: (**a**) Branching chorionic villi as viewed grossly in saline with magnification. (**b**) Histologic appearance of normal first trimester villi with nonspecific involutional changes; focal hyalinization and hypovascularity (40×). (**c**) Histologic appearance of dysmorphic villi suggestive of chromosomal abnormalities with irregular contour, trophoblast inclusions, and villous trophoblast sprouts (40×). (**d**) Chronic histiocytic intervillositis with normal villi and a dense monomorphic infiltrate of maternal monocyte-macrophages in the intervillous space (100×)

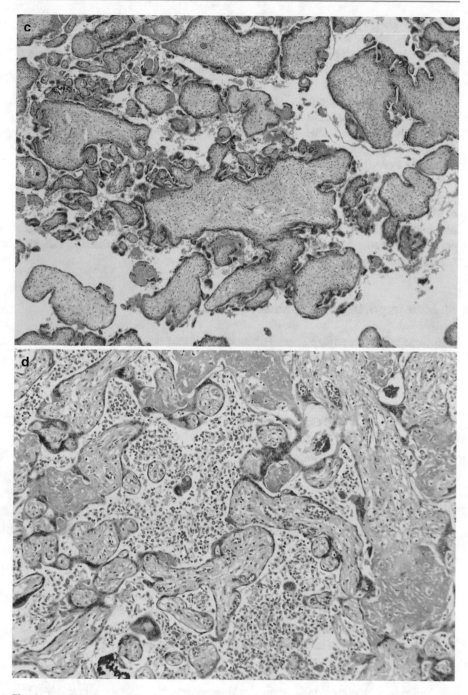

Fig. 1 (continued)

In general, specimens, especially from so-called complete or missed abortions (see above), can be adequately evaluated with three sections; one of villous tissue (the bisected remaining half of any specimen submitted for cytogenetic analysis if performed), one of decidualized endometrium, and one with a mix of tissues, including areas of blood clot and necrosis. Specimens with grossly cystic villi (greater than 2 mm maximum diameter) should have 2–3 additional cassettes submitted to rule out gestational trophoblastic disease. In cases without obvious villous tissue, submitting the entire specimen may be considered in the interest of rapid diagnosis to prevent clinical complications such as ruptured ectopic pregnancy. If trophoblast or villi are not identified by microscopy after the initial sampling, the entire remaining specimen is submitted and the clinician notified that an intrauterine pregnancy cannot be confirmed. Specimens grossly consisting entirely of clotted blood are a special case. They should be pulled apart to identify areas suggestive of entrapped tissue and a maximum of six sections submitted. Further sampling is generally unproductive and clinicians need to use clinical judgement to guide subsequent management.

Specific Important Histopathologic Sequences

Before describing specific placental phenotypes, it may be useful to review the common involutional changes that provide no additional information regarding pathogenesis, karyotype, or recurrence risk [4, 5] (Fig. 1b). The earliest such degenerative change is focal karyorrhexis of villous endothelium and circulating fetal blood cells. Next, fluid begins to accumulate in the villous stroma causing focal edema (hydropic change). Finally, after longstanding fetal death, the villi become fibrotic (hyalinized) with gradual loss of fetal vessels (hypovascular or avascular villi).

1. *Uniformly hydropic avascular villi consistent with anembryonic pregnancy*:
   This distinct sequence is characterized by an early-mid first trimester chorionic sac, generally without evidence of amnion, yolk sac, umbilical cord, or fetal tissue that shows uniformly hydropic villi without villous capillaries and lacks any distinction between proximal and distal villi. From a conceptual standpoint, it is useful to consider hydropic change as representing continuing trophoblast fluid transport in the absence of any fetal capacity to take up and excrete fluid. These histopathologic findings correlate with the absence of an embryonic pole by early ultrasound. While occasionally misdiagnosed as molar pregnancies by ultrasonography based on the degree of hydropic change, these cases lack any evidence of trophoblast hyperplasia by pathologic examination. Approximately 50% of specimens in this category have an abnormal karyotype [4].
2. *Diffuse intervillous hemorrhage (Breus' mole)*
   This relatively uncommon phenotype is defined by an early first trimester chorionic sac with normal villi, often showing nonspecific involutional changes, in a background of diffuse expansion of the intervillous space by recent hemorrhage. Pathogenesis is unproven, but may relate to failure of normal "plugging" of the

spiral arteries by endovascular extravillous trophoblast leading to the unimpeded entry of high pressure arterial blood into the fragile early intervillous space leading to disruption. Some think this lesion forms a continuum with massive subchorial thrombohematoma, a lesion occurring at later stages of pregnancy (see below) [6]. Karyotype is often normal in pregnancies with this phenotype.

3. *Dysmorphic villi suggestive of chromosomal abnormality*:

Dysmorphic villous features can be separated into two groups, circumferential trophoblast hyperplasia and abnormal villous architecture [4, 7, 8]. Villi with non-circumferential (polar) trophoblast hyperplasia usually originate from near the cytotrophoblast shell and can be discounted. A specific type of non-circumferential villous trophoblast hyperplasia, excessive trophoblast sprouting characterized by numerous thin filiform projections of syncytiotrophoblast projecting into the intervillous space, often occurs together with abnormal villous architecture (see below) and is commonly seen with monosomy X and other chromosomal abnormalities.

Circumferential villous trophoblast hyperplasia is associated with specific chromosomal abnormalities: diandric diploidy (complete hydatidiform mole), diandric triploidy (partial hydatidiform mole), and trisomies 7 and 15 (nonspecific trophoblast hyperplasia). Detailed discussion of these entities is beyond the scope of this chapter and the reader is referred to other more specific sources [7, 9]. In brief, complete moles show diffuse hyperplasia of both cytotrophoblast and syncytiotrophoblast and are accompanied by a monomorphic population of molar villi without other abnormal architectural features while partial moles show only focal-patchy hyperplasia involving predominantly syncytiotrophoblast, contain a dimorphic population of small and large villi, and manifest most of the abnormal villous architectural features described below. Of note, some cases of a rare lesion known as mesenchymal dysplasia (discussed below) may include small foci of complete mole with trophoblast hyperplasia, reflecting the diandric nature of both processes [10, 11]. Trisomies 7 and 15 and other conceptuses with nonspecific trophoblast hyperplasia generally lack abnormal villous architecture. As a general rule, any case with trophoblast hyperplasia should be followed by at least one interval maternal hCG titer to ensure return to baseline.

Abnormal villous architecture is defined by one or more of the following features: irregular villous contour (jagged, fjord-like invaginations or blunt cauliflower-like branching), villous stromal trophoblastic inclusions, abnormal villous capillary vascular pattern, and excessive trophoblast sprouts (Fig. 1c). Abnormal architecture without trophoblast hyperplasia is highly specific for chromosomal abnormalities [8], but the following caveats are important: (1) focal or borderline changes are nonspecific and should not be reported and (2) most chromosomal abnormalities do not show dysmorphic features (low sensitivity).

4. *Chronic thrombo-inflammatory lesions*:

This term covers a spectrum of partially overlapping lesions including diffuse perivillous fibrin(oid) deposition, chronic histiocytic intervillositis, and chronic decidual perivasculitis with lymphoplasmacytic deciduitis [5]. Contrary to the above group, these lesions are associated with a normal karyotype (high specificity, low sensitivity). Importantly, they have a high recurrence risk and are most commonly seen in cases of recurrent early pregnancy loss. Diffuse perivillous fibrin deposition ("maternal floor infarction") is another important cause of recurrent early trimester loss that can overlap histologically with chronic histiocytic intervillositis at this stage of pregnancy [12, 13]. However, because it more frequently presents at a later stage of pregnancy it is discussed in detail below.

Chronic histiocytic intervillositis is defined as a diffuse infiltration of the intervillous space by monomorphic CD68 positive monocyte-macrophages without a prominent lymphocytic component and without accompanying chronic villitis [14] (Fig. 1d). Although sometimes occurring at later stages of pregnancy, unlike maternal floor infarction, this lesion is most common in the first trimester. Recurrence rate is very high, approaching 70% in some studies [15]. Recent successful treatment using corticosteroids and aspirin has been reported in a small number of patients [16].

Chronic decidual perivasculitis with *lymphoplasmacytic deciduitis* is characterized by mural hypertrophy of decidual arterioles with a perivascular chronic inflammatory infiltrate in a background of well-preserved gestational endometrium with numerous plasma cells (chronic endometritis) [5]. In some cases, frank small vessel arteritis may be seen. In the personal experience of one author (RR), the most common clinical association is with recurrent pregnancy loss in patients with subclinical or overt autoimmune disease.

Pathology report: The convention we use at our institution for early fetal stage specimens without recognizable fetal anomalies is to provide two diagnoses (Fig. 2). The first describes the developmental stage of the chorionic sac (early mid or late first trimester), non-chorionic structures including fetal tissue with its state of preservation, umbilical cord, yolk sac, and amnion, and ending by describing the villi (morphology, vascularity, and/or involutional change) and intervillous space (inflammation, fibrin deposition, and/or expansile hemorrhage). The second describes the gestational endometrium and implantation site; well preserved versus necrotic, hemorrhagic, and/or any inflammatory infiltrates.

Representative pathology report: first trimester fetus and placenta

---

PRODUCTS OF CONCEPTION:
--LATE FIRST TRIMESTER CHORIONIC SAC WITH AUTOLYZED FETAL TISSUE, UMBILICAL CORD, FUSED AMNIO-CHORION, AND DYSMORPHIC VILLI SUGGESTIVE OF CHROMOSOMAL ABNORMALITY
--WELL PRESERVED GESTATIONAL ENDOMETRIUM AND IMPLANTATION SITE

NOTE: Villi show abnormal contour, trophoblast inclusions, and an abnormal capillary vascular pattern. Dimorphic populations of small and large villi, molar villi, and trophoblast hyperplasia are not observed excluding partial hydatidiform mole.

Fig. 2 First trimester placental pathology report

References

1. Langston C, Kaplan C, Macpherson T, et al. Practice guideline for examination of the placenta. Arch Pathol Lab Med. 1997;121:449–76.
2. Cox P, Evans C. Tissue pathway for histropathologic examination of the placenta. Royal College of Pathologists: London; 2017.
3. Kidron D, Bernheim J, Aviram R. Placental findings contributing to fetal death, a study of 120 stillbirths between 23 and 40 weeks gestation. Placenta. 2009;30:700–4.
4. Redline RW, Zaragoza MV, Hassold T. Prevalence of developmental and inflammatory lesions in non-molar first trimester spontaneous abortions. Hum Pathol. 1999;30:93–100.
5. Redline RW. Early pregnancy loss with normal karyotype. In: Redline RW, Boyd TK, Roberts DJ, editors. Placental and gestational pathology. Cambridge: Cambridge University Press; 2018. p. 9–15.
6. Shanklin DR, Scott JS. Massive subchorial thrombohaematoma (Breus' mole). Br J Obstet Gynaecol. 1975;82:476–87.
7. Redline RW, Hassold T, Zaragoza MV. Determinants of trophoblast hyperplasia in spontaneous abortions. Mod Pathol. 1998;11:762–8.
8. Redline RW. Early pregnancy loss with abnormal karyotype. In: Redline RW, Boyd TK, Roberts DJ, editors. Placental and gestational pathology. Cambridge: Cambridge University Press; 2018. p. 16–20.
9. Banet N, Descipio C, Murphy KM, et al. Characteristics of hydatidiform moles: analysis of a prospective series with p57 immunohistochemistry and molecular genotyping. Mod Pathol. 2014;27:238–54.
10. Hoffner L, Dunn J, Esposito N, et al. P57KIP2 immunostaining and molecular cytogenetics: combined approach aids in diagnosis of morphologically challenging cases with molar phenotype and in detecting androgenetic cell lines in mosaic/chimeric conceptions. Hum Pathol. 2008;39:63–72.
11. Lewis GH, DeScipio C, Murphy KM, et al. Characterization of androgenetic/biparental mosaic/chimeric conceptions, including those with a molar component: morphology, p57 immnohistochemistry, molecular genotyping, and risk of persistent gestational trophoblastic disease. Int J Gynecol Pathol. 2013;32:199–214.
12. Kim EN, Lee JY, Shim J-Y, et al. Clinicopathologic characteristics of miscarriages featuring placental massive perivillous fibrin deposition. Placenta. 2019;86:45–51. https://doi.org/10.1016/j.placenta.2019.07.006.
13. Weber MA, Nikkels PG, Hamoen K, et al. Co-occurrence of massive perivillous fibrin deposition and chronic intervillositis: case report. Pediatr Dev Pathol. 2006;9:234–8.
14. Doss BJ, Greene MF, Hill J, et al. Massive chronic intervillositis associated with recurrent abortions. Hum Pathol. 1995;26:1245–51.
15. Boyd TK, Redline RW. Chronic histiocytic intervillositis: a placental lesion associated with recurrent reproductive loss. Hum Pathol. 2000;31:1389–92.
16. Mekinian A, Costedoat-Chalumeau N, Masseau A, et al. Chronic histiocytic intervillositis: outcome, associated diseases and treatment in a multicenter prospective study. Autoimmunity. 2015;48:40–5.

Late Fetal Stage (Previable) Placenta (Second Trimester, 12–22 Weeks Post LMP)

Raymond W. Redline and Sanjita Ravishankar

Adverse Outcomes/Clinical Presentations

- Early stillbirth
- Late miscarriage/previable preterm birth
  - Vaginal bleeding/abruption
  - Preterm premature rupture of membranes
  - Cervical insufficiency
- Indicated termination for fetal anomalies or severe maternal disease
- Recurrent late miscarriage

Approach to the Gross Specimen

Gross specimens from this stage of pregnancy show the most heterogeneity ranging from "completely fragmented" in earlier cases to an intact fetus and placenta in later cases. Restricting this discussion to the placenta, it is important to weigh placental tissue trimmed of umbilical cord and membranes for comparison to normal reference values (Table 1); attempt to ascertain the location and nature of the umbilical cord insertion site; describe any cystic, solid, or hemorrhagic lesions; and note any alterations in the color and consistency of the parenchyma, umbilical cord, and fetal surface. Despite the fragmented nature of some specimens, the general rules of sampling membranes, umbilical cord, full thickness parenchyma, and lesions with adjacent normal parenchyma apply (described in detail below for later specimens). In grossly unremarkable cases, three sections of placental tissue are usually sufficient.

R. W. Redline (✉) · S. Ravishankar
Perinatal, Pediatric, and Gynecologic Pathology, Case Western Reserve University School of Medicine, University Hospitals Cleveland Medical Center, Cleveland, OH, USA
e-mail: raymondw.redline@Uhhospitals.org

© Springer Nature Switzerland AG 2021
J. Martinovic (ed.), *Practical Manual of Fetal Pathology*,
https://doi.org/10.1007/978-3-030-42492-3_14

Table 1 Means and standard deviations for placental and fetal weights by gestational age (UH Cleveland Medical Center, 2006–2015, unpublished data)

Gestational Age range (weeks))		Placental Weight (g)		Birth Weight (g)
12–12.9	Mean	39		18
$N = 9$	(SD)	−42	$N = 12$	−5
13–13.9	Mean	44		28
$N = 35$	(SD)	−15	$N = 41$	−6
14–14.9	Mean	52		46
$N = 54$	(SD)	−22	$N = 57$	−11
15–15.9	Mean	63		69
$N = 33$	(SD)	−17	$N = 32$	−13
16–16.9	Mean	74		99
$N = 25$	(SD)	−18	$N = 25$	−12
17–17.9	Mean	81		125
$N = 20$	(SD)	−24	$N = 15$	−18
18–18.9	Mean	92		172
$N = 11$	(SD)	−17	$N = 11$	−25
19–19.9	Mean	121		229
$N = 6$	(SD)	−30	$N = 6$	−43
20–20.9	Mean	116		307
$N = 4$	(SD)	−23	$N = 4$	−27

Specific Important Histopathologic Sequences

1. *Marginal abruption, acute and/or chronic*

   The preponderance of large remodeled spiral arteries in the central 2/3 of the placenta biases venous drainage to the placental margins. Although earlier descriptions of a continuous draining venous sinus are erroneous, decidual veins at the placental margin (where the chorionic and basal plates come together to form the placental membranes) are typically dilated and poorly supported by surrounding connective tissue. This places them at high risk for rupture in cases of decidual inflammation, increased maternal venous pressure, or abrupt changes in intrauterine geometry after rupture of membranes [1]. Acute marginal abruption is a common cause of both second and early third trimester premature loss, often occurring in combination with rupture of membranes and acute chorioamnionitis. Chronic marginal abruption often begins in the first trimester with vaginal bleeding and sonographic evidence of so-called "subchorionic hemorrhage" [2]. These early subchorionic hemorrhages may either resolve spontaneously or progress. With progression, persistent vaginal bleeding and oligohydramnios (chronic abruption/oligohydramnios sequence), and a constellation of placental findings including circumvallate membrane insertion, green (biliverdin) discoloration, organizing marginal blood clots, and diffuse chorioamnionic hemosiderosis may be observed [3–5](Fig. 1a). Diffuse chorioamnionic hemosiderosis

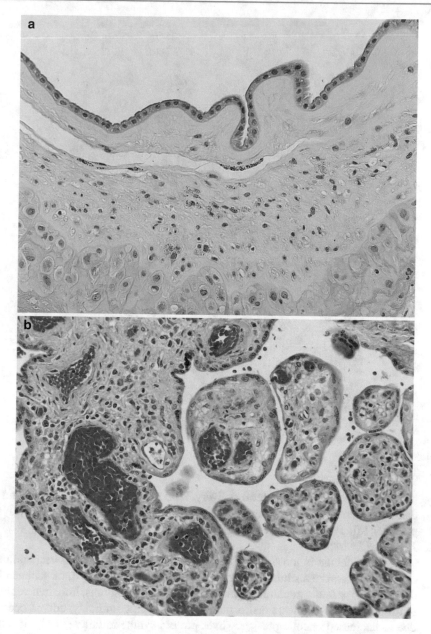

Fig. 1 Second trimester placental pathology: (**a**) Diffuse chorioamnionic hemosiderosis with numerous golden brown refractile hemosiderin crystals within the connective tissue of the chorion and amnion (200×). (**b**) Cytomegalovirus (CMV) villitis with villous stromal plasma cells on the left and large CMV nuclear inclusions on the right (200×). (**c**) Amnion Disruption Anterior Malformation (ADAM) sequence with absent umbilical cord, amnion disruption, and amnionic adhesions fusing the placenta to a fetus with an anterior wall defect. (**d**) Massive subchorial thrombohematoma with a large expansile hemorrhage elevating the chorionic plate above the underlying villous parenchyma

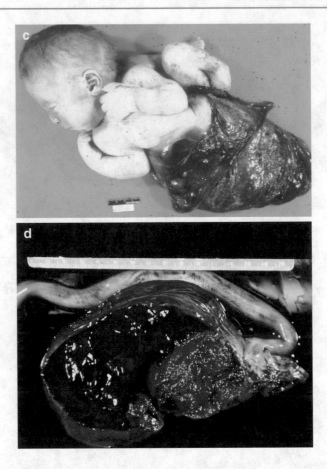

Fig. 1 (continued)

has been associated with preterm delivery, fetal growth restriction (FGR), and a distinct pattern of neonatal lung disease (so-called "dry" bronchopulmonary dysplasia or Mikity–Wilson disease) [6].

2. *Placental hydrops*

Hydrops fetalis is most commonly caused by fetal congestive heart failure due to either severe anemia (isoimmune, Parvovirus B19-related, or genetically determined) or fetal structural anomalies (arteriovenous shunts, impaired venous return, or right sided heart malformations) [7]. Less commonly, edema occurs due to decreased oncotic pressure (liver protein synthetic failure) or lymphatic malformations. Common gross and histologic findings in the placenta include increased weight for GA, pallor, villous edema, delayed villous maturation, and abnormalities at the villous trophoblast-stromal interface (artifactual cleavage and/or basement membrane calcification). The placenta plays a limited role in the differential diagnosis of hydrops. Presence or absence of increased circulating NRBC can broadly distinguish cases due to fetal anemia from other etiologies. In occasional cases, specific findings such as AV shunting in a large placental chorangioma, viral inclusions in Parvovirus B19 infection, and findings suggestive of TORCH infection or metabolic storage disease (see below) may be diagnostic.

3. *Chronic villitis, infectious ("TORCH infection")*

   Hematogenous infections of the placenta by specific bacteria (*Treponema pallidum*), protozoa (*Toxoplasma gondii, Trypanosoma cruzi*), and viruses (Zika virus and Herpes viridiae: cytomegalovirus (CMV), Varicella-Zoster, herpes simplex, Epstein Barr) typically evoke a lymphohistiocytic inflammatory response in the placental villi known as chronic villitis [8, 9]. These infections, together with some no longer seen in the developed world (Rubella, Vaccinia, Variola), are grouped under the acronym TORCH (Toxoplasmosis, Other, Rubella, CMV, and Herpes simplex). The most common of these infections in Europe and North America is CMV. Typical features of infectious villitis that distinguish it from the much more common, and later occurring, noninfectious villitis (see below) include diffuse but variable involvement of most villi, a predominance of histiocytes over lymphocytes, fetal endothelial damage with stromal hemosiderin, villous stromal and endovascular fibrosis, calcification, delayed villous maturation, and, in some cases, villous plasma cells and/or viral inclusions (both most commonly seen in CMV) (Fig. 1b). Typical histopathology, immunohistochemical staining, and evidence of fetal infection allow for definitive diagnosis in most cases. Prognosis for the pregnancy and fetus vary according to the causative organism but early miscarriage, FGR, stillbirth, and organ-specific malformations, deformations, and disruptions are all possible sequelae. Extent and severity of placental involvement generally parallel the severity of fetal disease.

4. *Amnion adhesions/premature amnion rupture*

   Defects in the formation and integrity of the amnion straddle the boundaries of malformation, deformation, and disruption. In the earliest presentation, the amniotic deformities, adhesions, and mutilation (ADAM) sequence are thought to be secondary to dysmorphogenesis of the body stalk with associated short umbilical cord, failure of abdominal wall closure, and amnionic adhesions fusing the placenta to the developing fetus [10, 11] (Fig. 1c). Later, isolated amnion rupture can lead to the formation of amnionic bands that can encircle and amputate fetal body parts or encircle and constrict the umbilical cord (disruptions) [12]. In the placenta, amnion rupture may be diagnosed grossly by string-like amnion bands connecting the surface of the chorionic plate to the UC or histologically as separation of the amnion from the chorion with degenerating and/or calcified amniotic epithelial cells between the two membrane layers. Finally, amnion and chorion can rupture together without triggering labor (prolonged preterm rupture of membranes) leading to loss of amniotic fluid and an increased risk for the fetal oligohydramnios deformation sequence (Potter syndrome) and ascending bacterial/fungal infections (discussed below). Amnion nodosum, defined by organized nodules of degenerating fetal squamous cells incorporated into the amnionic epithelium, is a specific placental lesion associated with prolonged rupture of membranes, longstanding oligohydramnios, and lethal pulmonary hypoplasia.

5. *Massive subchorial thrombohematoma*

Large, expansile subchorionic hemorrhages that distort and elevate the chorionic plate (Fig. 1d) are rare lesions with a very high rate of associated stillbirth [13]. At one time they were thought to be a consequence of fetal death, but case reports of liveborns disproved this hypothesis. Pathogenesis is unknown. Parallels with diffuse intervillous hemorrhage (Breus' mole, see above), subchorionic intervillous thrombi, and excessive subchorionic fibrin have all been drawn, but are not entirely satisfactory. Three possible scenarios are (1) overexpansion of the intervillous space due to inadequate villous support related to distal villous hypoplasia and a thick "jelly-like" placenta by ultrasound, (2) early intraplacental abruptions analogous to the recently described infarction-hematoma (discussed below), and (3) hemorrhage due to stem villous rupture with both fetal hemorrhage and secondary maternal thrombosis.

Pathology Report

The pathology report from a second trimester loss should separately address the fetus and placenta. In most cases of sporadic loss related to placental disease, the fetus lacks specific abnormalities aside from fragmentation due to the method of evacuation, involutional changes caused by antenatal fetal death, and growth abnormalities related to maternal-placental dysfunction. Accordingly, the first line of a typical diagnostic report can be outlined as follows (Fig. 2): *fragmented/intact, autolyzed/well preserved, (male/female) fetus/fetal fragments; small for/large for/ appropriate for ___ weeks gestation by measurements; no congenital anomalies.* In most cases, the placental findings can be summarized in a second diagnostic line outlined as: *markedly fragmented/(complete/incomplete)/(relatively small/relatively*

Representative pathology report: second trimester fetus and placenta

---

FETUS AND PLACENTA:
--AUTOLYZED 125 G MALE FETUS; SMALL FOR 18 WEEKS
  GESTATIONAL AGE
--NO CONGENITAL ANOMALIES

--FRAGMENTED (?INCOMPLETE) SECOND TRIMESTER PLACENTA; 80 G
  IN AGGREGATE
--MASSIVE SUBCHORIAL THROMBO-HEMATOMA

NOTE: Massive subchorial thrombo-hematoma is a rare idiopathic expansile intraplacental hemorrhage often associated with fetal death. Recurrence risk is unknown.

Fig. 2 Second trimester placental pathology report

*large) intact second trimester placenta, ___ g (in aggregate), with...*Any specific placental diagnoses are then listed in order of importance followed by a note correlating the antenatal history and the fetal and placental findings with pathogenesis, risk of recurrence, and any suggestions for further diagnostic evaluation.

References

1. Harris BA. Peripheral placental separation: a review. Obstet Gynecol Surv. 1988;43:577–81.
2. Tuuli MG, Norman SM, Odibo AO, et al. Perinatal outcomes in women with subchorionic hematoma: a systematic review and meta-analysis. Obstet Gynecol. 2011;117:1205–12.
3. Elliott JP, Gilpin B, Strong TH Jr, et al. Chronic abruption-oligohydramnios sequence. J Reprod Med. 1998;43:418–22.
4. Naftolin F, Khudr G, Benirschke K, et al. The syndrome of chronic abruptio placentae, hydrorrhea, and circumallate placenta. Am J Obstet Gynecol. 1973;116:347–50.
5. Redline RW, Wilson-Costello D. Chronic peripheral separation of placenta: the significance of diffuse chorioamnionic hemosiderosis. Am J Clin Pathol. 1999;111:804–10.
6. Yoshida S, Kikuchi A, Sunagawa S, et al. Pregnancy complicated by diffuse chorioamniotic hemosiderosis: obstetric features and influence on respiratory diseases of the infant. J Obstet Gynaecol Res. 2007;33:788–92.
7. Machin GA. Hydrops revisited: literature review of 1,414 cases published in the 1980s. Am J Med Genet. 1989;34:366–90.
8. Altshuler G, Russell P. The human placental villitides: a review of chronic intrauterine infection. Curr Top Pathol. 1975;60:63–112.
9. Bittencourt AL, Garcia AG. The placenta in hematogenous infections. Pediatr Pathol Mol Med. 2002;21:401–32.
10. Yang SS. ADAM sequence and innocent amniotic band: manifestations of early amnion rupture. Am J Med Genet. 1990;37:562–8.
11. Opitz JM, Johnson DR, Gilbert-Barness EF. ADAM "sequence" partII: hypothesis and speculation. Am J Med Genet. 2015;167A(3):478–503.
12. Jacques S, Qureshi F. Early and late amnion rupture/amnion rupture and amnion nodosum. In: Redline RW, Boyd TK, Roberts DJ, editors. Placental and gestational pathology. Cambridge: Cambridge University Press; 2018. p. 214–9.
13. Shanklin DR, Scott JS. Massive subchorial thrombohaematoma (Breus' mole). Br J Obstet Gynaecol. 1975;82:476–87.

Early Preterm Placenta (Early Third Trimester: 23–32 Weeks)

Raymond W. Redline and Sanjita Ravishankar

Adverse Outcomes/Clinical Presentations:

- Fetal growth restriction (FGR)
- Stillbirth, often with FGR
- Spontaneous preterm delivery
  - Premature labor
  - Preterm premature rupture of membranes
  - Vaginal bleeding/abruption
  - Cervical insufficiency
  - Ascending bacterial/fungal infection
- Indicated preterm delivery
  - Fetal or maternal distress
  - Fetal anomalies: malformations, genetic/chromosomal disorders
- Twin transfusion syndrome
- Recurrent early preterm delivery/stillbirth

Approach to the Gross Specimen

Singleton placentas: The general approach to all placentas delivered after 23 weeks (early preterm, late preterm, and term) is similar and described in detail here. The completeness of the basal plate is assessed and possibly incomplete specimens are documented in the final diagnostic report to alert clinicians to the risks of morbidly adherent (accreta spectrum) or retained placenta; both of which can lead to postpartum hemorrhage, subsequent infertility, and recurrence. Sections taken near the

R. W. Redline (✉) · S. Ravishankar
Perinatal, Pediatric, and Gynecologic Pathology, Case Western Reserve University
School of Medicine, University Hospitals Cleveland Medical Center, Cleveland, OH, USA
e-mail: raymondw.redline@Uhhospitals.org

© Springer Nature Switzerland AG 2021
J. Martinovic (ed.), *Practical Manual of Fetal Pathology*,
https://doi.org/10.1007/978-3-030-42492-3_15

interface of normal and torn parenchyma are best for detecting foci of accreta. Abnormal shapes (accessory lobes, multilobation, irregular contour, or decreased width relative to length) are documented as they signify abnormal development and can also result in ectopic fetal vessels traveling within the membranes that are at risk for disruption (ruptured vasa previa, see below). Umbilical cord abnormalities including marginal/membranous insertion, furcate or tethered insertion, hypercoiling/stricture, or excessive length are important because of their relationship to fetal vascular malperfusion. Circumvallate (non-peripheral) membrane insertion may in some cases be associated with chronic abruption. Following complete examination and in selected cases photographic documentation of these abnormalities, two sections of umbilical cord and two sections of peripheral placenta with membranes rolled around them are obtained and the cord and membranes removed from the disc. The trimmed placenta is then weighed to determine weight and fetoplacental weight ratio for gestational age relative to standard reference tables (Table 1). Finally, serial "bread loaf" sectioning of the parenchyma is performed searching for firm lesion, cysts, and hemorrhages. Representative sections from each type of lesion are then submitted to demonstrate both the lesion and its surrounding parenchyma. In addition to the umbilical cord and membrane rolls, we always submit at least three parenchymal sections, one taken at the umbilical cord insertion site.

Placentas from multiple gestations: The approach to twin and higher order multiple placentas varies according to the number of chorions and amnions separating each pair. Dichorionic placentas, both separate and fused, have an opaque three-layered dividing membrane. They are divided, separately weighed, and processed as described above for singletons. Gross findings such as weight, shape, umbilical cord anatomy, and/or parenchymal lesions may help explain discordant fetal growth in some cases.

A monochorionic placenta, on the other hand, either lacks or has a translucent two-layered dividing membrane composed of the fused amnions from the two amniotic cavities without any intervening chorionic tissue. Once the nature of the dividing membrane has been determined by gross examination, a monochorionic placenta is treated as one for the purpose of measurements (weight, length, width, thickness) and the approximate percentage of the fetal surface occupied by each twin is estimated based on the relative distribution of chorionic vessels on the fetal surface. Insertion sites of both umbilical cords, both relative to the nearest margin and with respect to one another are measured. The fetal surface is inspected for surface artery-artery and vein-vein anastomoses. If the monochorionic placenta is intact without history or stillbirth, injection of the fetal vessels to document deep arteriovenous anastomoses is attempted. A quick method is to select the thinner umbilical cord (usually the donor in a twin-twin transfusion scenario, see below) and then sequentially inject the 3–5 major chorionic arteries (arteries pass over veins) with air using a large syringe looking for veins in the opposite twin's vascular territory that contain air bubbles. If anastomoses are not found, the arteries from the second twin are injected in a similar fashion. More rigorous methods using dye or contrast injections are usually restricted to a research setting and will not be described here. The placentas of triplets and higher order multiple gestations can show a mixture of

Table 1 Means and standard deviations for placental weights and dimensions, birth weights, and fetoplacental weight ratios by gestational age (UH Cleveland Medical Center, 2006–2015)

Gestational Age range (weeks)		Placental Weight (g)	Length/maximum Diameter (cm)	Breadth/minimum Diameter (cm)	Length minus Breadth (cm)	Calculated Average thickness (cm)		Birth Weight (g)	Fetoplacental Weight ratio
23–23.9 N = 42	Mean	157	14.8	11.8	3	1.2	N = 20	583	4
	(SD)	–43	–2.6	–1.6	–2.5	–0.3		–131	–1.5
24–24.9 N = 51	Mean	172	14.4	12.1	2.2	1.3	N = 24	665	4.3
	(SD)	–63	–2	–2	–1.9	–0.5		–86	–1
25–25.9 N = 63	Mean	181	14.9	12.5	2.4	1.3	N = 37	764	4.6
	(SD)	–71	–2	–1.9	–2.1	–0.4		–123	–1.2
26–26.9 N = 56	Mean	194	15.5	13	2.5	1.3	N = 36	840	4.5
	(SD)	–56	–2.5	–1.9	–1.9	–0.3		–206	–1.3
27–27.9 N = 45	Mean	202	14.9	13	1.9	1.3	N = 17	940	4.8
	(SD)	–62	–1.8	–2.1	–1.6	–0.3		–265	–1.1
28–28.9 N = 77	Mean	246	16.1	13.6	2.5	1.5	N = 48	1159	4.9
	(SD)	–70	–2.3	1.9)	–1.7	–0.4		–245	–1.3
29–29.9 N = 76	Mean	248	16	13.6	2.3	1.5	N = 40	1336	6.1
	(SD)	–80	–2.1	–1.9	–1.6	–0.5		–505	–3.8
30–30.9 N = 106	Mean	297	17.1	14.8	2.3	1.6	N = 69	1540	5.7
	(SD)	–118	–2.6	–2.3	–1.9	–1.2		–383	–1.7
31–31.9 N = 104	Mean	286	17	14.6	2.5	1.5	N = 67	1595	5.8
	(SD)	–74	–2.5	–2.1	–1.8	–0.3		–370	–1.3
32–32.9 N = 152	Mean	319	17.5	15.1	2.5	1.5	N = 107	1894	6
	(SD)	–82	–2.1	–1.8	–1.8	–2.1		–433	–1.4
33–33.9	Mean	348	17.9	15.4	2.5	1.6		2033	6.1

(continued)

Table 1 (continued)

Gestational Age range (weeks)		Placental Weight (g)	Length/maximum Diameter (cm)	Breadth/minimum Diameter (cm)	Length minus Breadth (cm)	Calculated Average thickness (cm)		Birth Weight (g)	Fetoplacental Weight ratio
N = 194	(SD)	-95	-2.4	-2	-2	-0.4	N = 130	-392	-1.3
34–34.9	Mean	377	18.4	15.8	2.6	1.7		2232	6
N = 335	(SD)	-88	-2.4	-2	-2.1	-0.4	N = 261	-400	-1
35–35.9	Mean	403	18.6	16	2.6	1.7		2447	6.3
N = 375	(SD)	-102	-2.5	-2.1	-2.6	-0.4	N = 328	-440	-1.4
36–36.9	Mean	419	19.2	16.4	2.8	1.7		2687	6.6
N = 515	(SD)	-106	-0.4	-2.1	-2.6	-0.4	N = 465	-462	-1.3
37–37.9	Mean	430	19.2	16.6	2.7	1.8		2908	6.9
N = 552	(SD)	-110	-2.7	-2.3	-2.5	-0.4	N = 497	-585	-1.4
38–38.9	Mean	434	19.4	16.7	2.8	1.7		3063	7.3
N = 1053	(SD)	-109	-2.5	-2.2	-2.4	-0.5	N = 944	-507	-2.4
39–39.9	Mean	460	19.7	17	2.8	1.8		3219	7.2
N = 1406	(SD)	-151	-2.6	-2.1	-2.3	-0.5	N = 1257	-503	-1.6
40–40.9	Mean	481	20	17.3	2.7	1.8		3405	7.3
N = 1249	(SD)	-131	-2.6	-2.2	-2.3	-0.8	N = 1094	-459	-1.2
41–41.9	Mean	495	20.4	17.4	3	1.8		3508	7.4
N = 497	(SD)	-109	-2.9	-2.3	-2.9	-0.4	N = 450	-463	-3

dichorionic and monochorionic relationships with one another. Each relationship should be documented by assessment of the corresponding dividing membranes, appropriate measurements, and performance of injection studies as indicated. Photographic documentation of the fetal surface in the fresh state should be archived to allow retrospective analysis if needed.

Specific Important Histopathologic Sequences

1. *Acute chorioamnionitis*

   Bacterial/fungal infection of the placental membranes is the most common pathologic process seen in cases of early preterm delivery but is not infrequent at earlier and later stages of pregnancy. The overwhelming majority of these infections are caused by organisms, either native to or colonizing the vagina, that ascend through the cervix, cross the placental membranes, and proliferate in the amniotic fluid. Organisms in the amniotic fluid elicit an acute maternally derived inflammatory response that emanates from decidual venules in the membranes and maternal blood in the intervillous space. Neutrophils enter the chorionic connective tissue (maternal stage 1) and progress to the amnion (maternal stage 2) eventually causing necrosis of the amnionic epithelium (maternal stage 3) [1, 2] (Fig. 1a). A concomitant acute fetally derived inflammatory response (usually present) begins in the walls of chorionic vessels and/or the umbilical vein (fetal stage 1), progresses to involve one or both umbilical arteries (fetal stage 2), and eventually spreads into the Wharton's jelly of the umbilical cord where it becomes organized in an arc-like distribution around the umbilical vessels (fetal stage 3). In rare cases, organisms may infect the placental membranes by hematogenous seeding during episodes of bacteremia, such as those that occur with severe maternal periodontal disease [3]. The dual placental inflammatory responses (acute chorioamnionitis), together with the epithelial barriers to fetal infection in the fetal lung and GI tract, are effective defense mechanisms preventing all but the most aggressive organisms (e.g., group B streptococci, enteric bacilli, Listeria monocytogenes) from causing fetal sepsis and death. The cost to the pregnancy is activation of the innate immune system often resulting in myometrial contractions and preterm delivery. Since the adaptive immune system at the maternal-fetal interface is normally downregulated preventing complete resolution of the infection, this triggering of labor may represent an evolutionary mechanism to maximize survival of mother and infant.

2. *Maternal vascular malperfusion*

   Successful human pregnancy depends on the ability of fully differentiated extravillous trophoblast to deeply invade the decidua and inner third of the myometrium and actively remodel the maternal spiral arteries. Remodeling entails both replacement of the vascular smooth muscle by fibrinoid matrix and luminal dilatation facilitating the flow of maternal blood into the intervillous space [4]. The complex pathophysiology that results in incomplete differentiation of extravillous trophoblast, shallow implantation, and failure to adequately remodel

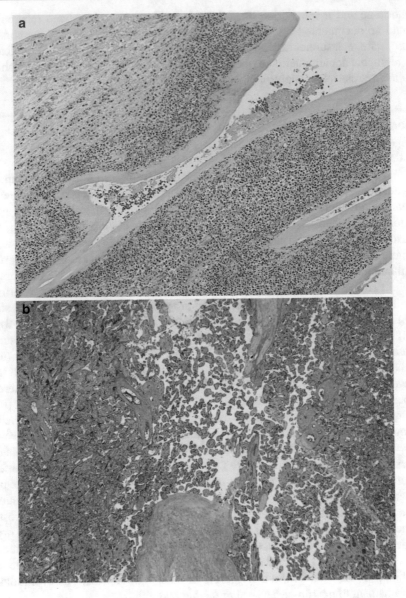

Fig. 1 Early third trimester placental pathology: (**a**) Necrotizing chorioamnionitis (maternal stage 3) with amnionic epithelial cell necrosis, abundant degenerating maternal neutrophils, and a bright red discoloration of the amnionic basement membrane (100×). (**b**) Accelerated villous maturation secondary to maternal vascular malperfusion. Preterm placenta shows alternating areas of crowded villi with villous agglutination and increased syncytial knots and areas of villous paucity with focal distal villous hypoplasia (20×). (**c**) Infarction-hematoma (rounded intervillous hematoma). Basally oriented, central hemorrhage with a rim of infarcted villi believed to represent an intraplacental abruption developing secondary to spiral artery rupture (20×). (**d**) Diffuse perivillous fibrin(oid) deposition ("maternal floor infarction") with normally spaced villi surrounded by a mixture of fibrin and fibrinoid matrix material in a lace-like distribution affecting most of the distal villi in at least 25% of the total placental parenchyma (40×)

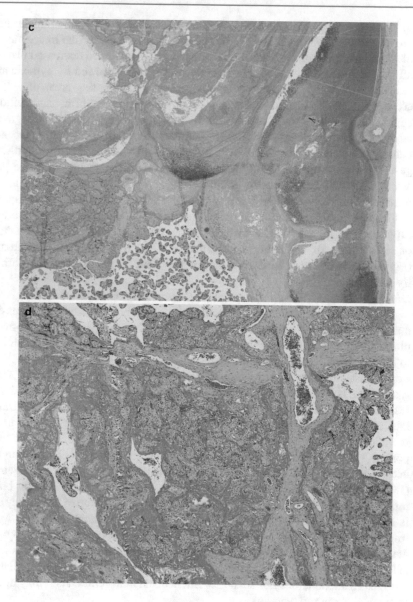

Fig. 1 (continued)

the spiral arteries is not yet fully understood, but is thought to involve underlying vascular disease, genetic risk factors, and dysregulated maternal-fetal interactions [5]. Maternal factors increasing risk include nulliparity, African ancestry, diabetes, atherosclerosis, essential hypertension, obesity, chronic renal disease, and autoimmune disease. Risk is also increased in pregnancies with an excessive total volume of placental trophoblast (e.g., twin pregnancy, hydatidiform mole, and placentomegaly).

There are two important late consequences of shallow implantation and failure of spiral artery remodeling [2, 6]. The first is maternal vascular malperfusion of the intervillous space. When global or partial, this results in decreased placental weight and accelerated villous maturation, a process caused by hypoxia and oxidative stress and characterized histologically by alternating areas of villous crowding with increased syncytial knots, intervillous fibrin, and villous agglutination and paucity due to villous hypoplasia [7] (Fig. 1b). When segmental and complete, it leads to villous infarction with loss of functioning placental parenchyma. Both forms of maternal vascular malperfusion are associated with gestational hypertension, FGR, spontaneous preterm labor, and indicated preterm delivery. The second important complication of abnormal spiral artery remodeling is rupture due to weakening of the vessel wall either by vasospasm with ischemia-reperfusion or fibrinoid necrosis (acute atherosis). Spiral artery rupture results in extensive hemorrhage, either retroplacental (abruptio placenta) or intraplacental (infarction-hematoma/rounded intraplacental hematoma) (Fig. 1c). Associated adverse outcomes include severe fetal or maternal morbidity and death.

3. *Diffuse perivillous fibrin(oid) deposition ("maternal floor infarction")*

This idiopathic placental reaction pattern is characterized by excessive amounts of fibrin and fibrinoid matrix that surround a large proportion (30–50%) of the villi in the inner lower two-thirds of the placenta [8, 9] (Fig. 1d). Contrary to the term "infarction," ischemic changes are not prominent. Rather the villous trophoblast atrophies, villi remain separated from one another, and, in some cases, there is an increase in extravillous trophoblast. One hypothesis is that this lesion represents an epithelial-mesenchymal transformation of villous to extravillous trophoblast triggered by one of a variety of severe insults that results in the secretion of excessive amounts of trophoblast-derived extracellular matrix components such as oncofetal fibronectin and type IV collagen [10]. This lesion has been associated with fetal Long-Chain 3-Hydroxyacyl-CoA Dehydrogenase (LCHAD) deficiency, accelerated hypertension, and early viral infections, but is most commonly unexplained [11–13]. It can occur at any stage of pregnancy and is associated with a high risk of pregnancy loss and neonatal morbidity. Most importantly, it has a high recurrence risk (up to 50% in some series) so appropriate genetic counseling and close monitoring of subsequent pregnancies is indicated. Furthermore, recurrent MFI can be observed in stillborns in an association with fetal skeletal anomalies such as shortened and bent femurs, and may mimic some fetal chondrodysplasias.

4. *Findings consistent with genetic/metabolic disease*

Most common inherited errors of metabolism do not have a placental phenotype and lesions suggestive of specific disorders are uncommon. However, rapid identification and communication of suggestive findings can be critical for the timely treatment of affected neonates. Suggestive findings fall into two categories [14]. First is lysosomal storage disease (LSD) [15]. Five specific LSD are associated with diffuse vacuolation of villous and extravillous trophoblast, ammonic epithelium, and villous Hofbauer cells by excessive amounts of mucopolysaccharides: galactosialidosis, sialidosis, infantile sialic acid storage disorder, I-cell disease, and GM-1 gangliosidase deficiency. Wolman disease shows similar vacuolation, in this case due to intracellular lipid, and Type IV glycogen storage disease shows polyglucosan inclusions restricted to extravillous trophoblast alone [16]. While Hofbauer cells in some other types of LSD may show specific diagnostic findings by EM, they are indistinguishable from normal by light microscopy [17]. The second category is fetal Bartter syndrome [18]. Placentas in this condition show patchy-diffuse villous trophoblast basement membrane calcification in the absence of predisposing clinical conditions (hydrops, stillbirth, or aneuploidy) or other associated pathologic lesions (maternal or fetal vascular malperfusion). While not as specific as the findings indicative of LSD, this pattern of calcification can be an important etiologic clue in cases of renal dysfunction in the context of polyhydramnios and fetal electrolyte abnormalities.

5. *Fetal vascular complications of monochorionic twin pregnancies*

Understanding the anatomic basis and clinical consequences of vascular anastomoses in monochorionic twin placentas has advanced considerably over the past 20 years [19, 20]. The prototypical disorder, chronic twin transfusion syndrome (TTS), is caused by major deep arteriovenous anastomoses, often associated with a paucity of balancing surface arterio-arterial anastomoses. The term chronic TTS is now restricted to cases with very early discordant fetal growth associated with severe oligohydramnios in the presumed donor twin and polyhydramnios in the presumed recipient. This imbalance can be aggravated by anatomic crowding of the donor to a restricted segment of the uterus, further impairing its perfusion (so-called "trapped twin"). Without laser ablation of the causative anastomoses, most of these cases will result in death or other severe adverse outcomes for both twins. A second disorder, twin anemia polycythemia syndrome (TAPS), occurs later in pregnancy when imbalances in vascular anastomoses lead to a more sudden transfusion of blood from one twin to the other. TAPS, equally as TTS caused by usually small AVA, is characterized by unequal umbilical cord diameters, villous edema in the recipient, and an increase in circulating fetal NRBC in both twins. One important subtype of TAPS is the sudden circulatory shift that occurs following the death of one twin in utero leading to hypotension and severe CNS damage in the survivor. A third disorder, twin reversed arterial perfusion (TRAP), can occur when there is a single major arterio-arterial anastomosis located between closely apposed umbilical cords in monochorionic twins. Early imbalances in perfusion pressure, sometimes due to congenital malformation, lead to persistently reversed flow in the umbilical and iliac arteries resulting in gradual involution of the upper body including the cardiovascular system of the affected, so-called "acardiac twin."

Pathology Report

Placentas from singleton pregnancies: Our philosophy is to keep reports as short and simple as possible for clarity while at the same time using consistent and precise terminology that allows us to retrieve details such as relative maturity, size for gestational age, grade and stage of the specific important pathologic sequences, and other important contributing diagnoses later for investigational purposes. Placentas are not tumors where many specific details and measurements are critical for clinical management, so we do not employ synoptic reporting. Likewise they are not autopsies where many disparate data elements must be weighed, so we do not routinely write long detailed comments. Instead we rely on defining the specific clinical questions to be addressed, reporting results promptly and succinctly, and following up with clinical colleagues when indicated to guide interpretation and management on a case by case basis.

Specifically, our reports are structured as described below and illustrated in Fig. 2. The first line conveys the following information: intact versus fragmented (?incomplete), placental weight with identification of relatively small or large placentas (less than 10th or greater than 90th centile for GA), abnormal coloration (e.g., brown, green, yellow), and the observed villous maturity independent of the actual GA (categories: immature—typical for 23–32 weeks, slightly immature—typical for 32–37 weeks, and mature—typical for 38–41 weeks). Subsequent lines list major pathologic sequences with appropriate grading, staging, and the individual supportive findings. Additional lines are added if necessary for any "accessory" findings that are less likely to have affected outcome.

Placentas from multiple pregnancy: Reports of placental pathology from multiple gestations follow the same general outline described above for singleton placentas. Additional specific aspects of these reports are described below and illustrated in Fig. 3. Dichorionic twin placentas are described as either separate or fused, weights for each after separation are recorded, and deviation from the 10 to 90th

---

Representative pathology report: third trimester singleton placenta

---

PLACENTA:
--RELATIVELY SMALL, MATURE PLACENTA
        (340 GMS; LESS THAN 1OTH PERCENTILE FOR 37 WEEKS).
--CHRONIC VILLITIS, HIGH GRADE, DIFFUSE, WITH STEM VESSEL
  OBLITERATION AND EXTENSIVE AVSCULAR VILLI
--INCREASED CIRCULATING FETAL NUCLEATED RED BLOOD CELLS

NOTE: High grade chronic villitis with obliterative vascular changes has been associated with neonatal encephalopathy, as was seen in this case.
Increased circulating fetal nucleated red blood cells in the absence of fetal hemorrhage are consistent with significant hypoxia of at least 6-12 hours duration. Recurrence risk is estimated at 20-50%.

Fig. 2 Third trimester singleton placental pathology report

Representative pathology report: monochorionic twin placenta

TWIN PLACENTA:
--RELATIVELY SMALL, IMMATURE MONOCHORIONIC DIAMNIONIC TWIN
 PLACENTA (310 GMS; LESS THAN 10TH PERCENTILE FOR 28 WEEKS).
--DISCORDANT FEATURES: DECREASED UMBILICAL CORD DIAMETER;
 PALLOR AND DECREASED PARENCHYMAL SHARE, PLACENTA A
--DEEP ARTERIOVENOUS ANASTOMOSES TWIN A TO TWIN B
--PAUCITY OF SURFACE ARTERIO-ATERIAL ANASTOMOSES

NOTE: The placental features are all consistent with the clinical diagnosis of twin-twin transfusion syndrome with twin A as the donor and twin B as the recipient. Monochorionic twin placentas are almost invariably monozygous.

Fig. 3 Third trimester pathology report for placentas from multiple pregnancies

centile range of weight for gestational age is noted. A monochorionic twin placenta is never divided, but unequal percentages for the vascular territory on the chorionic plate are reported. Unlike singletons, our reports from the placentas of multiple pregnancies always include a note. The implications of the observed chorionicity for zygosity are explained (i.e., "zygosity cannot be assessed in dichorionic twins" and "monochorionic twins are almost invariably monozygotic"). Cases without proper labeling to designate twin of origin or in which the pathologic changes suggest that labeling may have been in error (e.g., chorioamnionitis in twin B only) are highlighted. Finally, any significantly discordant fetal growth (>25%) is discussed in terms of possible placental causes such as vascular anastomoses, peripheral UC insertion, or localized histopathologic abnormalities.

References

1. Redline RW, Faye-Petersen O, Heller D, et al. Amniotic infection syndrome: nosology and reproducibility of placental reaction patterns. Pediatr Dev Pathol. 2003;6:435–48.
2. Khong TY, Mooney EE, Ariel I, et al. Sampling and definitions of placental lesions: Amsterdam Placental Workshop Group Consensus Statement. Arch Pathol Lab Med. 2016;140:698–713.
3. Han YW, Fardini Y, Chen C, et al. Term stillbirth caused by oral Fusobacterium nucleatum. Obstet Gynecol. 2010;115:442–5.
4. Brosens I, Pijnenborg R, Vercruysse L, et al. The "Great Obstetrical Syndromes" are associated with disorders of deep placentation. Am J Obstet Gynecol. 2010;204:193–201.
5. Lain KY, Roberts JM. Contemporary concepts of the pathogenesis and management of preeclampsia. JAMA. 2002;287:3183–6.
6. Redline RW, Boyd T, Campbell V, et al. Maternal vascular underperfusion: nosology and reproducibility of placental reaction patterns. Pediatr Dev Pathol. 2004;7:237–49.
7. Cindrova-Davies T, Fogarty NME, Jones CJP, et al. Evidence of oxidative stress-induced senescence in mature, post-mature and pathological human placentas. Placenta. 2018;68:15–22.
8. Andres RL, Kuyper W, Resnik R, et al. The association of maternal floor infarction of the placenta with adverse perinatal outcome. Am J Obstet Gynecol. 1990;163:935–8.
9. Katzman PJ, Genest DR. Maternal floor infarction and massive perivillous fibrin deposition: histological definitions, association with intrauterine fetal growth restriction, and risk of recurrence. Pediatr Dev Pathol. 2002;5:159–64.

10. Redline RW. Invited Commentary—Maternal floor infarction and massive perivillous fibrin deposition: clinicopathologic entities in flux. Adv Anat Pathol. 2002;9:372–3.
11. Griffin AC, Strauss AW, Bennett MJ, et al. Mutations in long-chain 3-hydroxyacyl coenzyme a dehydrogenase are associated with placental maternal floor infarction/massive perivillous fibrin deposition. Pediatr Dev Pathol. 2004;15:368–74.
12. Redline RW, Jiang JG, Shah D. Discordancy for maternal floor infarction in dizygotic twin placentas. Hum Pathol. 2003;34:822–4.
13. Yu W, Tellier R, Wright JR Jr. Coxsackie virus A16 infection of placenta with massive perivillous fibrin deposition leading to intrauterine fetal demise at 36 weeks gestation. Pediatr Dev Pathol. 2015;18:331–4.
14. Redline RW. Lysosomal storage disease, Bartter syndrome, and mimics. In: Redline RW, Boyd TK, Roberts DJ, editors. Placental and gestational pathology. Cambridge: Cambridge University Press; 2018. p. 235–40.
15. Roberts DJ, Ampola MG, Lage JM. Diagnosis of unsuspected fetal metabolic storage disease by routine placental examination. Pediatr Pathol. 1991;11:647–56.
16. Dainese L, Adam N, Boudjemaa S, et al. Glycogen storage disease type IV and early implantation defect: early trophoblastic involvement associated with a new GBE1 mutation. Pediatr Dev Pathol. 2016;19:512–5.
17. Fowler DJ, Anderson G, Vellodi A, et al. Electron microscopy of chorionic villus samples for prenatal diagnosis of lysosomal storage disorders. Ultrastruct Pathol. 2007;31:15–21.
18. Maruyama H, Shinno Y, Fujiwara K, et al. Nephrocalcinosis and placental findings in neonatal bartter syndrome. AJP Rep. 2013;3:21–4.
19. Lewi L, Deprest J, Hecher K. The vascular anastomoses in monochorionic twin pregnancies and their clinical consequences. Am J Obstet Gynecol. 2013;208:19–30.
20. De Paepe ME, Burke S, Luks FI, et al. Demonstration of placental vascular anatomy in monochorionic twin gestations. Pediatr Dev Pathol. 2002;5:37–44.

Late Preterm/Term Placentas (Late Third Trimester: 32–42 Weeks from LMP)

Raymond W. Redline and Sanjita Ravishankar

Adverse Outcomes/Clinical Presentations:

Hypoxic-ischemic encephalopathy/Neonatal encephalopathy
Stillbirth (IUFD)
Intrapartum death
Fetal growth restriction (FGR)
Fetal anomalies
Recurrent late pregnancy loss

Approach to the Gross Specimen

The general approach to placentas delivered after 23 weeks was outlined in the previous section and only a few points of emphasis pertaining to findings most relevant to adverse outcomes in late preterm and term placentas will be mentioned here. The first is the identification of an umbilical cord at risk for interrupted fetoplacental blood flow. Relevant findings include abnormal cord insertion (see below), deformations due to entanglements or prolapse, excessive cord length, hypercoiling, and true umbilical cord knots. The second is documentation of green discoloration of the membranes, chorionic plate, and sometimes the surface of the umbilical cord. Usually due to meconium staining, this finding should prompt histologic evaluation for the duration of meconium exposure. Finally, identification of excessively pale and/or edematous parenchyma that can accompany massive fetomaternal hemorrhage with or without superimposed hydrops fetalis.

R. W. Redline (✉) · S. Ravishankar
Perinatal, Pediatric, and Gynecologic Pathology, Case Western Reserve University School of Medicine, University Hospitals Cleveland Medical Center, Cleveland, OH, USA
e-mail: raymondw.redline@Uhhospitals.org

© Springer Nature Switzerland AG 2021
J. Martinovic (ed.), *Practical Manual of Fetal Pathology*,
https://doi.org/10.1007/978-3-030-42492-3_16

Specific Important Histopathologic Sequences

1. *Fetal vascular malperfusion/umbilical cord accidents*

   Impairment of fetal placental blood flow is the most frequent cause of still-birth and fetal brain injury during the latter stages of pregnancy [1, 2]. Sudden complete cessation of flow due to prolonged complete umbilical cord occlusion (e.g., acute umbilical cord prolapse) is a rare sentinel event leading to fetal death if not immediately relieved. Survivors generally lack long-term sequelae or die in the early neonatal period, although a small number will have devastating neurologic injuries. Partial prolonged compression or intermittent complete occlusion of umbilical vessels (subacute and/or chronic) is much more common, causing fetal vascular stasis within the placenta and, in some cases, fetal thromboembolic disease [3]. Abnormalities associated with reduced umbilical blood flow include (1) primary abnormalities at the junction of umbilical cord and placenta such as membranous insertion, loss of Wharton's jelly prior to insertion (furcate umbilical cord), or tethering of the umbilical cord by a tight fold of amnion from the chorionic plate, (2) secondary abnormalities such as hypercoiling, true knot, stricture, or increased resistance due to excessive cord length, and (3) extrinsic entanglements such as cord loops around the fetal neck or body (e.g., tight nuchal cord) or subacute cord prolapse following prolonged rupture of membranes. Other contributing factors include fetal cardiac insufficiency, polycythemia, hypercoagulability, and platelet disorders.

   Significant impairment of fetoplacental blood flow leads to a sequence of changes, collectively termed fetal vascular malperfusion, that affect all levels of the fetal placental circulation [4]. Increased fetal venous pressure and stasis can lead to thrombosis, luminal dilatation, and intramural fibrin deposition within the large fetal vessels of the chorionic plate and stem villi. Intermediate sized vessels may contract and develop bridging fibrosis culminating in luminal obliteration. However, degenerative changes in the distal villous tree are the most reliable indicators of fetal vascular malperfusion. Early lesions include necrosis of endothelial and stromal cells with extravasation of fetal red blood cells (villous stromal vascular karyorrhexis). In later lesions, villous capillaries disappear and the stroma becomes fibrotic resulting in contiguous clusters of hyalinized avascular villi. Umbilical cord compression without thrombosis is associated with scattered small foci of affected villi (<5 per focus) while stem vessel thrombosis leads to segmental malperfusion and much larger foci of affected villi (Fig. 1a). The most extreme example of fetal vascular malperfusion is the complete postmortem circulatory stasis accompanying stillbirth. These nonspecific diffuse changes seen in all stillborns must be distinguished from specific, patchy antemortem fetal vascular changes that may have contributed to death. Definitive diagnosis in this situation requires identification of large vessel lesions (thrombi, intramural fibrin, venous dilatation) and/or distinct regional differences in villous degenerative changes (focal hyalinized avascular villi). While recurring factors such as inherited thrombophilic mutations, platelet disorders, or antiphospholipid antibody syndrome may contribute in rare cases, the most

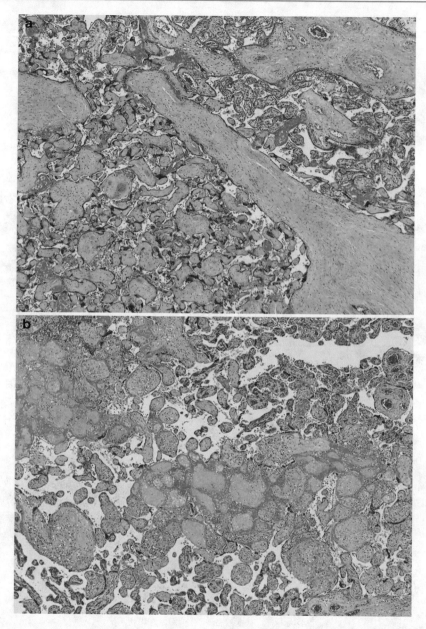

Fig. 1 Late third trimester placental pathology: (**a**) Fetal vascular malperfusion, segmental type, with a large contiguous focus of hyalinized avascular villi indicative of an upstream fetal thrombosis (40×). (**b**) Diffuse high grade chronic villitis (VUE) with multiple contiguous villi with lymphocytic infiltrates occupying at least 10% of total parenchyma plus numerous avascular villi with perivillous fibrin (40×). (**c**) Delayed villous maturation with enlarged terminal villi with increased stromal connective tissue, numerous centrally located capillaries, a thickened cellular layer of villous trophoblast, and a lack of vasculosyncytial membranes (100×). (**d**) Meconium-associated myonecrosis with rounded, discohesive peripheral vascular smooth muscle cells showing a pyknotic nucleus and glassy bright eosinophilic cytoplasm (200×)

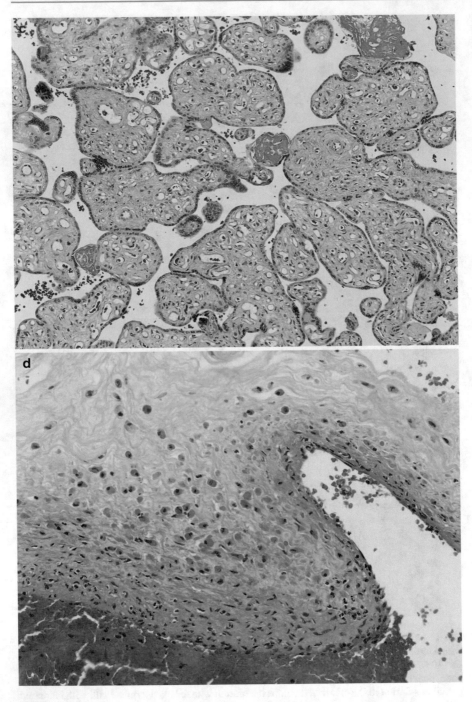

Fig. 1 (continued)

important conclusion applicable to most cases of fetal vascular malperfusion is that it reflects an umbilical cord accident unlikely to recur in subsequent pregnancies.

2. *Chronic villitis, noninfectious ("villitis of unknown etiology")*

   Chronic inflammation within the villous stroma is a feature shared by TORCH infections and so-called villitis of unknown etiology (VUE). Unlike TORCH infections (discussed above), VUE is a sharply circumscribed, T-cell predominant, inflammatory process affecting almost exclusively term or late preterm placentas [5, 6]. While infection can never be entirely excluded in cases of VUE, the absence of maternal or fetal infectious signs or symptoms, the lack of B lymphocytes and plasma cells, the maternal origin of the infiltrating T lymphocytes, distinct maternal serum cytokine and villous RNA expression profiles typical of allograft rejection, and the high recurrence rate all suggest an alloreactive maternal anti-fetal immune response mounted by maternal T lymphocytes against fetal antigens expressed on fetal cells in the villous stroma [7, 8]. Multiple levels of protection have evolved to protect the fetus from rejection, including absence of MHC antigens on trophoblast, local T regulatory cells, and ineffective local antigen presentation [9]. A potential breech in these defenses is introduced by focal erosions in the villous trophoblast barrier that allow maternal immune cells to gain access to unprotected fetal tissues. VUE is believed to be the result of this mixing of maternal and fetal cells.

   Chronic villitis (VUE) is usually low grade (less than ten affected villi per focus) or patchy high grade (greater than ten villi per focus) [10]. Additional histologic features such as involvement of more than 10% of all villi (diffuse VUE), extensive perivillous fibrin, large foci of avascular villi, and obliterative stem villous vasculopathy all significantly increase the risk of FGR, CNS injury, and stillbirth (Fig. 1b). Chronic villitis/VUE has a high recurrence rate (20–33%), so close early monitoring of subsequent pregnancies is indicated.

3. *Fetal stromal vascular abnormalities*

   Adaptive or developmental alterations in the villous architecture of late pregnancy can indicate genetic, epigenetic, or metabolic abnormalities. Most are not primary causes of fetal injury, but they can be associated with decreased placental efficiency and serve as biomarkers for environmental stressors affecting the pregnancy.

   Delayed villous maturation, sometimes called "maturation defect" or "distal villous immaturity," is characterized by a villous architecture more typical of an early preterm placenta and includes features such as increased stroma, more central fetal capillaries, a thickened excessively cellular layer of villous trophoblast, and paucity of vasculosyncytial membranes [10–12] (Fig. 1c). These features are most frequently seen in diabetic pregnancies with placentomegaly and may in this situation reflect a lack of terminal differentiation due to continuing villous growth. However, they can also be seen in smaller placentas associated with idiopathic IUFD at term, FGR, fetal vascular malperfusion, and resolved hydrops fetalis, so other factors may also be involved.

Villous capillary lesions may be separated into three subgroups, villous chorangiosis, placental chorangioma, and multifocal chorangiomatosis [13–15]. All have been associated with decreased maternal oxygen tension with an underlying maternal vascular malperfusion [16]. Etiologies include high altitude, smoking, anemia, high levels of air pollution, multiple gestation, and some cases of preeclampsia. Villous chorangiosis is limited to the distal villi and is defined by the finding of more than ten capillary cross sections per villus in ten or more contiguous villi at several different locations in the placenta. This lesion often accompanies other chronic villous pathology such as VUE, delayed villous maturation, and fetal vascular malperfusion. Placental chorangioma is a nodular tumor-like swelling within large stem villi and is composed of proliferating capillaries with prominent pericytes. Large chorangiomas can be associated with FGR, hydrops fetalis, and disseminated intravascular coagulation [17]. A rare, presumably genetic, process characterized by extremely large numbers of chorangiomas (multiple chorangioma syndrome) has been associated with recurrent stillbirth [18]. Multifocal chorangiomatosis is a more diffusely distributed proliferation of anastomosing capillaries that surround large muscularized fetal vessels in intermediate villi. Extensive multifocal chorangiomatosis has been associated with fetal malformations, idiopathic FGR, and Beckwith–Wiedemann syndrome.

Mesenchymal dysplasia is a rare developmental syndrome characterized by segmental vascular malformations, villous stromal overgrowth, and enlarged hydropic or molar villi [19, 20]. It is strongly associated with FGR and stillbirth [21]. While occasionally detected early in pregnancy, it is most commonly recognized at delivery or in late pregnancy as a partially cystic placenta by ultrasound. Most cases are mosaic for an androgenetic cell line (similar to complete hydatidiform mole) that spares the trophoblastic lineage and hence does not cause gestational trophoblastic disease (androgenetic biparental mosaic chimerism/ABMC) [22]. Some cases are associated with Beckwith–Wiedemann syndrome [23].

4. *Fetal hemorrhages*

Fetal hemorrhages can be separated into two subgroups; acute disruptions of large fetal vessels and massive fetomaternal hemorrhages [24, 25].

Large vessel hemorrhages usually occur during parturition in structurally abnormal placentas and involve unprotected fetal vessels in the umbilical cord (e.g., membranous insertion site) or chorionic plate (vessels bridging the placenta and accessory lobes). When these vessels overlap the cervix, a diagnosis of ruptured vasa previa can be made. Other antenatal causes of major vessel hemorrhage include ruptured complete placenta previa, iatrogenic complications of invasive procedures such as cordocentesis, and umbilical cord ulceration due to prolonged exposure to meconium or gastric acid (fetal pyloric stenosis) [26, 27].

Massive fetomaternal hemorrhage (FMH) is the most severe example of a common process: focal rupture of a terminal villus with loss of small amounts of fetal blood that is rapidly arrested by maternal coagulation triggered by exposed fetal collagen. This sequence results in placental lesions termed intervillous thrombi. Delay or failure to "seal off" these foci of hemorrhage can lead to massive FMH. Unsurprisingly, large or multiple intervillous thrombi increase the risk of significant blood loss. Other placental findings typical of massive FMH include marked villous edema and increased nucleated red blood cells. Definitive diagnosis requires testing for fetal red blood cells in the maternal circulation by the Kleihauer–Betke method or flow cytometry. Massive FMH is a significant cause of stillbirth, neonatal encephalopathy, and idiopathic hydrops fetalis and appropriate testing should be performed in all such cases [28, 29].

5. *Meconium-associated vascular myonecrosis*

Release of fetal stool (meconium) into the amniotic fluid is a common vagal response to minor stress observed in up to 30% of term vaginal deliveries. This reflex is generally absent prior to 34 weeks and hence is sign of fetal maturity. Identification of meconium staining is not the primary responsibility of the pathologist, as it is clearly recognizable at parturition, has little clinical impact in most cases, and can be ambiguous in some placentas. Our policy is to look for histologic evidence of meconium release in all green-stained placentas, in all cases where a clinical history of meconium stained fluid is provided, and whenever the placental membranes show typical low power histologic features such as a poorly cohesive membrane roll, subamnionic edema, or amnionic epithelial degeneration. In these cases, we attempt to answer three questions: (1) are there any typical vacuolated pigment-laden maternal macrophages (absent in very early cases), (2) are such macrophages limited to the membranes (early) or are they seen within the deep connective tissue of the chorionic plate (later), and (3) is there evidence of associated tissue damage? The most common form of tissue damage is fetal vascular myonecrosis [27, 30, 31]. This uncommon lesion is caused by prolonged exposure of vascular smooth muscle cells (myocytes) at the periphery of large fetal umbilical or chorionic vessels to the caustic effects of bile acids leading to myocyte necrosis/apoptosis (Fig. 1d). It is usually accompanied by pigment-laden maternal macrophages in the chorionic vessel wall. Meconium-associated myonecrosis has been shown to be a biomarker for adverse outcomes in term and near-term pregnancies [32]. Risk factors include intact membranes, oligohydramnios, and duration of meconium exposure of greater than 48 h. An even rarer consequence of prolonged meconium exposure is transmural erosion of the vessel wall leading to rupture and fetal exsanguination.

Pathology Report

The diagnostic report for term and late preterm placentas does not differ from that described above for early preterm placentas.

Summary

As discussed in this chapter, assessment of placental growth, architecture, and histopathology can play an important role in understanding fetal well-being at all stages of pregnancy. In selected cases, it can provide specific diagnoses with treatment implications for mother or infant, predict recurrence risks, and guide the management of future pregnancies. However, these benefits can only be realized if the appropriate placentas are submitted to pathology with a relevant clinical history, evaluated in a timely manner by experts trained in perinatal pathology, and reported in a format understood by all key members of the health care team.

References

1. Chisholm KM, Heerema-McKenney A. Fetal thrombotic vasculopathy: significance in live-born children using proposed society for pediatric pathology diagnostic criteria. Am J Surg Pathol. 2014;39:274–80.
2. Redline RW. Cerebral palsy in term infants: a clinicopathologic analysis of 158 medicolegal case reviews. Pediatr Dev Pathol. 2008;11:456–64.
3. Redline RW. Clinical and pathological umbilical cord abnormalities in fetal thrombotic vasculopathy. Hum Pathol. 2004;35:1494–8.
4. Redline RW, Ravishankar S. Fetal vascular malperfusion, an update. APMIS. 2018;126:561–9.
5. Altshuler G, Russell P. The human placental villitides: a review of chronic intrauterine infection. Curr Top Pathol. 1975;60:63–112.
6. Redline RW. Villitis of unknown etiology: noninfectious chronic villitis in the placenta. Hum Pathol. 2007;38:1439–46.
7. Kim MJ, Romero R, Kim CJ, et al. Villitis of unknown etiology is associated with a distinct pattern of chemokine up-regulation in the feto-maternal and placental compartments: implications for conjoint maternal allograft rejection and maternal anti-fetal graft-versus-host disease. J Immunol. 2009;182:3919–27.
8. Myerson D, Parkin RK, Benirschke K, et al. The pathogenesis of villitis of unknown etiology: analysis with a new conjoint immunohistochemistry-in situ hybridization procedure to identify specific maternal and fetal cells. Pediatr Dev Pathol. 2006;9:257–65.
9. PrabhuDas M, Bonney E, Caron K, et al. Immune mechanisms at the maternal-fetal interface: perspectives and challenges. Nat Immunol. 2015;16:328–34.
10. Khong TY, Mooney EE, Ariel I, et al. Sampling and definitions of placental lesions: Amsterdam Placental Workshop Group Consensus Statement. Arch Pathol Lab Med. 2016;140:698–713.
11. Redline R. Distal villous immaturity. Diagn Histopathol. 2012;18(5):189–94.
12. Stallmach T, Hebisch G, Meier K, et al. Rescue by birth: defective placental maturation and late fetal mortality. Obstet Gynecol. 2001;97:505–9.
13. Ogino S, Redline RW. Villous capillary lesions of the placenta: distinctions between chorangioma, chorangiomatosis, and chorangiosis. Hum Pathol. 2000;31:945–54.
14. Bagby C, Redline RW. Multifocal chorangiomatosis. Pediatr Dev Pathol. 2010;14:38–44.
15. Benirschke K. Recent trends in chorangiomas, especially those of multiple and recurrent chorangiomas. Pediat Devel Pathol. 1999;2:264–9.
16. Soma H, Watanabe Y, Hata T. Chorangiosis and chorangioma in three cohorts of placentas from Nepal, Tibet and Japan. Reprod Fertil Devel. 1996;7:1533–8.
17. Amer HZ, Heller DS. Chorangioma and related vascular lesions of the placenta--a review. Fetal Pediatr Pathol. 2010;29:199–206.
18. Gallot D, Marceau G, Laurichesse-Delmas H, et al. The changes in angiogenic gene expression in recurrent multiple chorioangiomas. Fetal Diagn Ther. 2007;22:161–8.
19. Jauniaux E, Nicolaides KH, Hustin J. Perinatal features associated with placental mesenchymal dysplasia. Placenta. 1997;18:701–6.
20. Faye-Petersen OM, Kapur RP. Placental mesenchymal dysplasia. Surg Pathol Clin. 2013;6:127–51.
21. Pham T, Steele J, Stayboldt C, et al. Placental mesenchymal dysplasia is associated with high rates of intrauterine growth restriction and fetal demise: a report of 11 new cases and a review of the literature. Am J Clin Pathol. 2006;126:67–78.

22. Kaiser-Rogers KA, McFadden DE, Livasy CA, et al. Androgenetic/biparental mosaicism causes placental mesenchymal dysplasia. J Med Genet. 2006;43.187–92.
23. Armes JE, McGown I, Williams M, et al. The placenta in Beckwith-Wiedemann syndrome: genotype-phenotype associations, excessive extravillous trophoblast and placental mesenchymal dysplasia. Pathology. 2012;44:519–27.
24. de Almeida V, Bowman JM. Massive fetomaternal hemorrhage: Manitoba experience. Obstet Gynecol. 1994;83:323–8.
25. Swank ML, Garite TJ, Maurel K, et al. Vasa previa: diagnosis and management. Am J Obstet Gynecol. 2016;215:223 e1–6.
26. Ichinose M, Takemura T, Andoh K, et al. Pathological analysis of umbilical cord ulceration associated with fetal duodenal and jejunal atresia. Placenta. 2010;31:1015–8.
27. Altshuler G, Arizawa M, Molnar-Nadasdy G. Meconium-induced umbilical cord vascular necrosis and ulceration: a potential link between the placenta and poor pregnancy outcome. Obstet Gynecol. 1992;79:760–6.
28. Laube DW, Schauberger CW. Fetomaternal bleeding as a cause for 'unexplained' fetal death. Obstet Gynecol. 1982;60:649–51.
29. Biankin SA, Arbuckle SM, Graf NS. Autopsy findings in a series of five cases of fetomaternal haemorrhages. Pathology. 2003;35:319–24.
30. King EL, Redline RW, Smith SD, et al. Myocytes of chorionic vessels from placentas with meconium associated vascular necrosis exhibit apoptotic markers. Hum Pathol. 2004;35:412–7.
31. Redline RW. Meconium associated vascular necrosis. Pathol Case Rev. 2010;15(3):55–7.
32. Redline RW. Severe fetal placental vascular lesions in term infants with neurologic impairment. Am J Obstet Gynecol. 2005;192:452–7.

Index

© Springer Nature Switzerland AG 2021
J. Martinovic (ed.), *Practical Manual of Fetal Pathology*,
https://doi.org/10.1007/978-3-030-42492-3

Printed in the United States
by Baker & Taylor Publisher Services